THE MEDICAL
CARNIVALESQUE

THE MEDICAL CARNIVALESQUE

FOLKLORE AMONG PHYSICIANS

LISA GABBERT

INDIANA UNIVERSITY PRESS

This book is a publication of

Indiana University Press
Office of Scholarly Publishing
Herman B Wells Library 350
1320 East 10th Street
Bloomington, Indiana 47405 USA

iupress.org

Manufactured in the United States of America

First printing 2024

Cataloging information is available from the Library of Congress.

ISBN 978-0-253-07024-1 (hardback)
ISBN 978-0-253-07023-4 (paperback)
ISBN 978-0-253-07025-8 (ebook)

For the Bill Walshes and all the other doctors

CONTENTS

FOREWORD

ANTONIO SALUD II, MD, MA

Suffering is pervasive in medicine. Suffering is not only experienced by patients and their families but also by physicians who battle sickness, death, and decay. Many times we succeed; other times, we recognize that the people we care for are at their life's end, but never without some type of sacrifice. As a physician, I realized years ago that taking care of people gave my life meaning and purpose but that it also was quite brutal to me and my family. We doctors chose our profession, but we cannot predict how we will respond to the challenges of medicine. This was especially true in 2020 when COVID-19 challenged our understanding of what and how life and health care should be. We saw unprecedented death and suffering, often met with ignorance, incompetence, and apathy. As a result, we experienced frustration, disillusionment, and burnout. Like many physicians, I am trying to heal from the trauma I experienced from the pandemic. That healing process involves reevaluating my life in terms of what I have done in my work and seeking a more balanced, authentic, and genuine existence. I am grateful for Dr. Gabbert and her book as they have helped me reminisce and understand why and how I arrived at this moment. The work I did with Dr. Gabbert helped me navigate through times of fear, uncertainty, and lack of control, both professionally and personally.

One of the most difficult aspects of doctoring for me has been to reconcile my duty as a physician to treat patients with my duty as a physician to do no harm. As physicians-in-training, we are told to first do no harm (*primum non nocere*). That dictum shapes our training and practice. Yet we are constantly faced with a paradox (and in some ways, paradox is the basis of the medical carnivalesque), which is that, in order to care for our patients, we must treat them with therapies and interventions that may contradict that mandate. I recall a specific time in my training when I tried to reconcile this dilemma. One evening shift, I was caring for a patient with multiorgan system failure. My attending physician instructed me to continue to give medications and blood to ensure his heart would continue beating and his blood pressure would remain normal. Many physicians would have deemed the therapies and interventions as futile at that point. I was conflicted the whole night. The patient remained alive until the next morning. By the end of my shift, I was physically exhausted and emotionally torn on how to care for a patient who was not going to be "cured." I asked myself a very basic question: "Are we giving this patient a chance to recover, or are we just prolonging the patient's suffering?" Soon after my shift, I spoke with my mentor and recounted the night's events. He then asked me how my mother was doing. A bit taken aback, not understanding what his question had to do with my current situation, I replied that she was fine. My mother had been diagnosed with breast cancer, which had spread to her lymph nodes. After a difficult course of treatment, she had responded and survived. Knowing this, my mentor explained that the patients and families who allow us to continue treatment when we may think all is futile give us an opportunity to discover if all truly is "futile." This uncertainty is common in medicine and reminds us of the interplay between hope and despair, science and art, life and death. This moment illustrates the always-present question that we physicians ask ourselves: "When is enough enough?" The seeming absurdity or futility of certain current therapies may provide insight on what may eventually become fruitful. The uncertain present becomes possibly meaningful for the future.

The medical carnivalesque is an aspect of culture that is buried deep within the training and practice of medicine. Dr. Gabbert and I had many conversations as we crafted the concept of the medical carnivalesque in 2009. These conversations yielded a framework to acknowledge and understand what some people would call "the hidden curriculum"—those behaviors that are subconsciously taught and learned by way of shared experience. Those practices range from objectifying persons as objects to using gallows humor as defense mechanisms. How do we do no harm when our profession and our journey are fraught with sacrifice, self-denial, and moral injury? How do we move forward? This work that Dr. Gabbert and I created helped me understand the specific ways in which physicians live in a space of constant tension between self and other, family and patient, sanity and madness, hope and despair. In this light, Dr. Gabbert's book provides a transparent look and a palpable feel on how we are transformed into physicians after we are accepted into medical school. We strive for clinical competence and excellence, but we are placed in situations that are neither clear nor straightforward. In doing so, we discover the need for resiliency during times of intolerable suffering. The medical carnivalesque describes the suffering, along with burnout, moral injury, and even trauma experienced by providers and health care staff alike. Without a way to address these issues over time, such experiences can lead to isolation and helplessness. Within this framework, Dr. Gabbert delves into stories about physician suffering and tragedies and explains how humor, superstitions, and folk beliefs may help physicians find a sense of harmony and meaning in an uncertain and, at times, seemingly absurd world.

In the last decade and a half, I have used the concept of the medical carnivalesque in the development of programs geared toward healing medical professionals. One such program based heavily on the medical carnivalesque is The Pathos Project, founded by Yuri Maricich and Keri Oxley and further developed by myself and Dr. Dominic Vachon.[1] The Pathos Project offers a curriculum for undergraduate students and medical students that explores themes of suffering, professional development, and spirituality. The Pathos Project provides a safe harbor where individuals exposed to the hidden curriculum can explore uncomfortable thoughts and behaviors in order to reach understanding. A good physician has the traits of competency, consistency, and compassion, but great physicians embody the more nuanced traits of curiosity, humility, and vulnerability. This approach is the beginning of a new way of thinking about doctoring. Our metrics of success for The Pathos Project are how we deliberately teach physicians-in-training to solve the problems that are not addressed elsewhere. Honesty and courage are what is needed to help us to rediscover the connection and community that these COVID-19 years have severely challenged.

We are all broken, but in the spirit of *kintsugi*, the Japanese technique in which something that is already imperfect and seemingly irreparable is repaired, we repair what is broken in us in order to become strong, beautiful, and whole again. Dr. Gabbert and her work on the medical carnivalesque provides us with the tools to be curious and vulnerable, to let go of control, and to be present with the people around us. Perhaps more importantly, this book gives us permission to laugh at the world and at ourselves. After all, laughter is the best medicine.

Note

1. Director of the Hillebrand Center for Compassionate Care in Medicine at the University of Notre Dame, Indiana.

ACKNOWLEDGMENTS

This book has taken years to research and write, and some of the ideas are rooted in experiences and conversations going back decades. I unfortunately cannot remember everyone who has influenced this project over the years, but I am particularly grateful to the following people.

First and foremost, I would like to acknowledge my husband, Bill Walsh, who talked with me endlessly about this project and whose experiences in medicine directly informed this research. He has been an unending source of love and support, and without him, this project never would have gotten off the ground. I am also very grateful to my father-in-law, Dr. William Walsh, Sr. I listened to stories about his residency at Bellevue Hospital in New York during the 1960s for years before starting to write, and these stories, some of which are included, have been influential in my thinking about the training of doctors during the middle of the twentieth century.

I would also like to thank my family, particularly my children Quinn and Bridget, who have literally grown up with this project. My parents, Dan and Friede Gabbert, and my bonus parents, Nancy Walsh and Mike DeVito, were wonderfully patient and supportive. I love you all very much. My dad died while the book was in production. I love and miss him very much.

I am incredibly lucky to have amazing friends and colleagues both at Utah State University and across the country. You are all smart, funny, and wickedly insightful. I am particularly grateful to Christine Cooper-Rompato and Steve Siporin. Their friendship, acuity, and expertise have been invaluable, and I would not have been able to complete this manuscript without the many conversations about death, humor, end-of-life issues, and suffering that we had. In addition, Ona Siporin, Keri Holt, Jeannie Thomas, Lynne S. McNeil, Randy Williams, Shane Graham, Christie Fox, Afsane Rezaei, Ehsan Estiri, Phebe Jensen, Lisa Gilman, John Fenn, Andrew Kolovos, LuAnne Roth, Danielle Christiansen, Kate Holbrook, Eric Eliason, Juwen Zhang, Simon Bronner, and Keiko Wells all have been good friends and colleagues. I would like to specifically acknowledge the excellent work of my undergraduate research assistant Samantha Wallace. She knocked on my door one day wondering if I had a project she might help with. She was, and remains, a godsend.

The physicians and medical students who shared their stories are at the heart of this book. They are hardworking, brave, and insightful people to whom I am deeply indebted. I hope I have accurately represented their experiences and that the profession finds this book helpful. First among these is Dr. Antonio Salud II, with whom I first collaborated and who was gracious enough to write the foreword. Dr. Salud has been my most enthusiastic supporter. He has taken the concept of the medical carnivalesque in related, more practical, directions since we met, and I look forward to our future endeavors. I am also grateful to my lovely friend Dr. Mary Burris, who offered many insights and perspectives on various topics, medical and otherwise.

Money and time are always useful, and I humbly thank the Department of English and the College of Humanities, Arts, and Social Sciences at Utah State University for various forms of support, including sabbatical leave, subvention monies, and several Creative Activity and Research Enhancement awards. I am particularly grateful to the American Folklife Center/Library of Congress's Occupational Folklife Project, which granted me an Archie Green Fellowship during the 2019–2020 academic year to conduct oral histories of physicians.

Finally, I would like to thank the editors and staff at Indiana University Press who shepherded this project through the publication process. Y'all do a lot of heavy lifting. I very much appreciate the anonymous readers who reviewed the manuscript. Reviewing takes a lot of time, and the suggestions ultimately helped improve this book.

THE MEDICAL
CARNIVALESQUE

Introduction

Medicine and doctoring have been portrayed as funny since antiquity. The earliest examples may date to the New Comedy of classical Greece. One illustrative excerpt is from Menander's play *Aspis*, lines 299–464, in which a fake doctor speaks medical nonsense (Kazantzidis 2018, 29). British classical scholar Hugh Lloyd-Jones (1971, 187) additionally writes that "the Spartan antiquary Sosibius remarked that the comic doctor was a stock figure of the ancient Doric farce, and this specimen was not the only one in Attic comedy."[1]

Most commonly, physicians and medicine were targets of parody and satire, particularly in medieval Europe. At that time, medical academic studies did not include patient observation or practical experience, leading to the popular perception that university-trained physicians were educated people with little hands-on knowledge. "A Mirror for Fools," for example, is a "rollicking comic poem" written by the monk Nigel of Longchamps in the twelfth century that targets medicine and involves a burlesque prescription for an ass who wants a longer tail (Wallis 2010, 526). The physician in the late fourteenth-century *Canterbury Tales* has been argued by some critics to be a less-than-admirable character, "a striking example of medical fraud" (Robertson 1988, 137) who would have been funny to medieval audiences. He is a hypocrite who performs affected piety (Longsworth 1971, 227), quotes authorities to impress his patients, and is overly interested in profit from his apothecaries (Sprunger 1996). Similar examples lampooning physicians and academic medicine can be found throughout the early modern period.

In the contemporary world, much humor about medicine stems from physicians themselves. Physicians are often portrayed as witty in popular culture. CBS's television show *M*A*S*H* ran from 1972 to 1983 and then for years after as a rerun. It featured Captains "Hawkeye" Pierce and "Trapper" McIntyre in the 4077th Mobile Army Surgical Hospital (M*A*S*H) unit during the Korean War who engaged in ongoing comic dialogue. A more recent example is the television medical comedy *Scrubs*, which aired from 2001 to 2010 and targeted physicians and the medical establishment. The slapstick show was set in a teaching hospital and focused on the comic and oftentimes surreal lives of medical interns.

Real physicians also use humor in their work, whether in day-to-day interactions with patients, among themselves, online, or in their writings. One of the best-known medical novels of all time is Samuel Shem's (real name Stephen Bergman) *The House of God* ([1978] 2003), a biting satire that targeted the terrible working conditions of residents in large US research hospitals during the late 1960s and '70s and was based on his own experiences. Today physicians commonly share humorous expressions on the internet, with blogs, websites, and YouTube videos devoted to medical comedy. One popular website, *GomerBlog.com*, for example, is dedicated to "Earth's Finest Medical News." It is the medical equivalent of the *Onion*, a popular satirical news source that satirizes current events. One *GomerBlog* headline, for example, posted on December 21, 2020, during the middle of the COVID-19 epidemic, read, "Hospital Combats Physician Burnout with Mandatory Burnout Training," targeting hospital bureaucracy and ineptitude. Such sites are produced by physicians and physicians are the primary audience. The humor is esoteric, meaning that it is not intended for outsiders and can be difficult for outsiders to understand.

My question is: Why is medicine a fertile arena for the comic? Is there something inherently amusing about doctoring, which involves the serious issues of illness, disease, and death? My research led me to conclude that medicine is a fertile arena for the comic because medicine grapples with life, death, suffering, and the body, and the comic is a useful means of addressing such topics. I argue that the specific vein characterizing much medical humor is the *carnivalesque*, an ancient orientation in which themes of life, death, and the body are central. It is a lowbrow, body-oriented mode that addresses the core philosophical and existential issues with which medicine regularly deals.

The term *humor* as a description for the materials covered in this book, however, is complex (Marsh 2019). The root of the word humor is itself medical, stemming from the ancient humoral system of medicine attributed to Hippocrates. A humor referred to one of the four fluids of the body, identified as blood, phlegm, yellow bile, and melancholy, otherwise known as the "black bile" (Wickberg 1998). An additional anatomical meaning, used in the past and also today, refers to humor as the transparent semifluid substances that fill the eye. The ancient humors drew on elements of nature, and their proportion and constitution determined the health of a person. For hundreds of years, the goal of Western medicine was to keep the humors in proper balance, and over time, the term *humor* came to signify temperament.[2] It wasn't until much later that *humor* was associated with the comic, although interestingly one humor, the black bile, was associated with the pervasive laughter of madness (Zatta 2001, 537–538).

Folklorist Moira Marsh (2019, 214–15) suggests that scholars use the term *humor* as little as possible, instead identifying genres or terms that isolate a specific component in humorous communication processes, such as jokes, dialect stories, or tall tales in order to be more precise. The focus of this study, however, is not specific genres but rather the general informal talk that occurs "backstage" among physicians, an idea taken from Erving Goffman (1961) that refers to social interactions conducted away from the public eye. This talk occurs between physicians rather than in front of patients. It is an occupational shoptalk that is often funny or playful, consisting not only of specific genres of humor, such as jokes, but also a broader body of work-related folklore, including witticisms, proverbial sayings, apocryphal stories, legends, insults, and the like, much of which is comical. This backstage occupational folklore tends to elicit laughter, whether funny or not (see Eagleton 2019a). The term *folklore* itself refers to informal, traditionalized aspects of culture, beliefs, and ways of communicating among and between groups. Since there is no good word that encompasses this body of material, I use the terms humor, folklore, humorous folklore, and occupational folklore to refer to it; I also identify and discuss specific genres when appropriate.

The audience for this backstage talk is other physicians, who form what anthropologists call "joking relationships" within the workplace that allow humorous communication to emerge. Mahadev L. Apte (1985, 54) points out that in industrial societies, joking is voluntary and individual, and so joking can become the basis of acceptance into social groups and of identity. This is certainly true of physicians, who begin forming their identity as doctors in medical school, which is when playful speech first emerges. Such intraphysician communication reveals values, attitudes, and perspectives about the group.

There are, of course, many different styles of humor that exist in medicine, spanning exoteric, satirical jokes about physicians and medicine (such as those that have existed for centuries) to the humorous forms used by doctors themselves, which include feel-good Patch Adams–type "clown" behavior for working with children, humor used in physician-patient interactions, and potentially harmful or problematic jokes and sarcastic asides or comments.

Physician-to-physician humor can be dark, and typically it has been framed as gallows or black humor (Watson 2011, Thorson 1993). This is how I first approached it as well. It is true that humor used by physicians can be earthy and transgressive, stemming as it does from difficult work contexts. Gallows humor, or *Galgenhumor*, in its narrow definition is literally the humor of a condemned person on the gallows. Sigmund Freud considered it a high form of humor where one laughs at one's own fragility (Thorson 1993). Others note that gallows humor typically refers to jokes made about and by victims of oppression (Dundes and Hauschild 1983).[3] An early study of gallows humor in Nazi-occupied Czechoslovakia, for example, concluded that it was born out of "sad experiences accompanied by grief and sorrow" (Obrdlik 1942, 715) but boosted morale among the oppressed and therefore had a positive function. Others concur that gallows humor has a coping function (e.g., Thorson 1993).

The related term *black humor* is less clearly defined, although it is usually characterized as aggressive.[4] Literary scholar Max F. Schulz (1973) argues that black humor is realism forced to the extreme of metaphysical truth, while a dictionary definition of black humor states that it is a "'dark, disturbing and often morbid or grotesque mode of comedy' that trades in 'death, suffering, or other anxiety-inducing subjects'" (cited in Buehrer 2017, 29). According to this definition, black humor does not differ from other kinds of humor except in the topics it addresses (see also Brock 2008 for an overview in which black humor lacks clear definition). Folklorist Claire Schmidt (2017) uses the term *sick humor* (Dundes 1987) to describe humor among prison guards, noting that it helps people both do their job and not do their job.

Conceptualizing backstage medical humorous folklore as gallows humor, black humor, or sick humor, however, does not fully capture the depth and nuances encompassed by the term *carnivalesque*, which is taken from the work of literary scholar Mikhail Bakhtin. It refers to a comic aesthetic style known as grotesque realism that temporarily and symbolically upends official forms of power vis-à-vis the body. In a previously published article I coauthored with Dr. Antonio Salud II (2009), we coined the term *medical carnivalesque* to characterize the subversiveness, inversions, and resistance found in medical humor.[5] Drawing on published and mass mediated sources, we argued that the medical carnivalesque was a means by which the medical community tacitly acknowledged the absurdities of the modern medical project. In this book, I develop the idea of playful backstage talk as carnivalesque by illustrating that the themes, issues, and topics in this body of folklore correlate quite closely to the principal themes embedded in ancient forms of the carnivalesque as described by Bakhtin. These include life, death, the body, and the contingent nature of official doctrine and perceived truth. Death, for example, is a main theme in gallows and black humor but, when understood within a carnivalesque orientation, exists as part of a broader aesthetic and philosophical system that connects life to death through bodily imagery and laughter. And unlike gallows, black, or sick humor, a carnivalesque perspective ultimately is about renewal.

All humor is potentially subversive. Apte (1985) observes that a general characteristic of humor is the inversion of traditional hierarchies, while anthropologist Mary Douglas (1968), speaking of jokes specifically, states that they tilt toward uncontrol. She characterizes jokes as "anti-rites"—that is, unlike standard rites that impose order and harmony, jokes promote disorder and "do not affirm the dominant values, but denigrate and devalue" (369). What is particular to a carnivalesque orientation and makes it especially apropos for medicine is that it accomplishes disorder, subversion, and denigration vis-à-vis a grotesque, transgressive body and its various functions, such as eating, birthing, defecating, having sex, and dying. This body is explained in further detail in chapter 4. In doing so, the medical carnivalesque mirrors the ongoing and often transgressive social situations in which real physicians find themselves as they go about their work on actual patient bodies. Douglas explains that spontaneous jokes (that is, humorous utterances) mirror the social situation in which they occur, meaning that there is some kind of disruption of social structure in the ongoing social situation that the humorous utterance expresses. In medicine, physicians transgress social and cultural boundaries in their work on the body; this social situation is then expressed in transgressive, body-oriented carnivalesque folklore.

I further argue that suffering is an essential component of the medical carnivalesque (Gabbert 2020). Suffering and humorous folklore are inexorably interconnected in medical work contexts, although it is challenging to establish a direct correlation. The folklore that emerges in medicine is connected to extraordinarily difficult, complex work environments in which health care workers not only grapple with the existential nature of patient suffering but also perform work that induces suffering in themselves. The transgression of social and cultural boundaries in the service of medicine contributes to this suffering, meaning that suffering suffuses medicine well beyond immediate patient care. The overall argument of this book, then, is that backstage medical folklore is carnivalesque and that this medical carnivalesque is underpinned by a context of institutionalized, work-related suffering.

I first became aware that medicine had its own body of occupational folklore when I was in graduate school at Indiana University in the late 1990s and early

2000s. I was pursuing a combined PhD in folklore and American studies when my partner entered medical school at the same time. He recognized folklore and began bringing home examples from his classes and rotations. The earliest examples were the informal, traditional mnemonics that circulate among students to help them memorize medical information, part of the "hidden curriculum" in medicine and of which humor is a part (Goldman 2014, 12). Mnemonics by definition are designed to be memorable, and these definitely were because many of them were quite dirty and sexist. The mnemonics surrounding the cranial nerves are perhaps the most widely known. The twelve cranial nerves are:

I. Olfactory
II. Ophthalmic
III. Oculomotor
IV. Trochlear
V. Trigeminal
VI. Abducens
VII. Facial
VIII. Acoustic
IX. Glossopharyngeal
X. Vagus
XI. Sensory (Accessory)
XII. Hypoglossal

One common mnemonic for memorizing them is: "O, O, O, To Touch And Feel A Girl's Vagina, Ah Heaven!" This is, as Anne Skomorowsky (2014) wryly notes, infinitely more memorable to medical students than an older version: "On Old Olympus's Towering Tops, A Finn and German Viewed A Hop." Another associated mnemonic is: "Some Say Marry Money; But My Brother Says Big Boobs Matter Most," which helps students remember whether each cranial nerve is sensory, motor, or both. Both of these still circulated during the first decade of the twenty-first century.

Such folklore is sexist and juvenile. But the context in which such examples emerge is important. This includes not only the historically patriarchal and sexist orientation of organized medicine but also a context in which students learn to transgress boundaries with ease and in doing so have their own ideas and values rearranged. Medical students who learn and pass on sexist mnemonics, for example, are having significant, life-changing experiences outside the realm of anything imaginable by the general public. Skomorowsky (2014) explains: "In the first years of medical school, the student will discuss sexual functions with men old enough to be her grandfather, and perform digital [meaning finger, addition mine] rectal examinations to feel their prostate glands, and observe young women in childbirth and sew their torn vaginas in its aftermath. For some students, the first nude body they ever see will belong to a cadaver. Medical school confronts the student with the living and dead body and its sexuality. The student uses humor to make this tolerable." Physicians-in-training break every boundary and taboo imaginable with respect to the body. These transgressive acts eventually become normal for physicians, placing them in a kind of permanent state of liminality and ambivalence in which humor becomes important currency. And like all folklore, medical folklore is constantly updated. The newest memorable version of the mnemonic for those important cranial nerves is LGBTQ+ friendly: "On Occasion Oliver Tries To Anally Finger Various Guys. Vaginas Are History!" (Skomorowksy 2014). This updated mnemonic is itself transgressive, challenging the heteronormativity of earlier versions.

Doctors continue to use folklore as they go through their training, which, depending on their specialty, can last for ten or more years *after* medical school. Over the years, as my spouse moved through the difficult periods of residency and fellowship, I was struck by how much doctors talked about work when they were together, the kinds of stories they told, and the slang that was used. Much of this folklore was funny. They recounted apocryphal stories, personal experience narratives, and legends. They also recounted practical jokes (Marsh 2015). One surgeon, for example, sent me a video in which his anesthesiologist pretended to be a patient under sedation in the operating room. The surgeon scrubbed up and went near the bed to start operating. The "patient" suddenly sprang up, making the surgeon jump and generating laughter from everyone in the room, all of whom were in on the joke—and secretly recording it on their phones. Physicians also participate in roasts, and they use slang, aphorisms, and proverbs in their everyday speech. I also learned that physicians have a host of folk beliefs (ideas articulated or purported but not necessarily believed) about good and bad luck at work.

Some physicians even compose and sing songs about work. These materials have become more readily available to the public as doctors post their performances on social media. Early studies of occupational folklore focused on singing in male working-class occupations that had traditions of balladry and work songs, such as mining, farming, timbering, and ranching (Koch 2012). Such songs were valuable because the lyrics, tune, function, and rhythm revealed much about people's feelings, values, and attitudes toward work (Groce 2019). In later years, protest songs and laborlore became an important focus

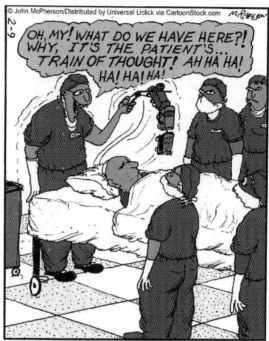

Every year or so, neurosurgeon Brian Baker
liked to pull the same stupid gag on
his colleagues.

Figure I.1. Cartoon illustrating medical work prank.

(e.g., Green 1987; McCarl 2006; Leary 2013). I have sometimes wondered jestingly to myself whether doctors might have been a focus of these early studies if they sang ballads.[6] Doctors don't sing ballads, but one colleague told me about a physician she knew who sometimes sang to premature babies, and I am sure this is not an isolated case. More frequently, younger doctors sing (and sometimes dance) *about* work on YouTube and TikTok, performances that parody workplace situations and poke fun at hospitals, other doctors, work hours, bureaucracy, and other aspects of medical life (Gabbert 2018). One of the most well-known physician-based singing groups in the 2000s was a British band called the Amateur Transplants who parodied well-known pop music tunes. A more recent example includes a parody of the well-known Disney song "Let It Go" from the movie *Frozen* and performed by students from the University of Chicago Pritzker School of Medicine as "I Don't Know" (see chap. 5).

Studies of physician-based occupational folklore cross a broad range of disciplines and have, like this one, largely focused on forms of humorous folk speech and verbal forms of interaction (for an exception that focuses on customs, see Hufford 1989). Many scholars have drawn on release and superiority theories of humor, arguing that folklore among physicians relieves stress or anxiety, acts as a defense mechanism, and expresses hostility toward patients (Coombs et al. 1993; Parsons et al. 2001). One well-known article is by folklorists Victoria George and Alan Dundes (1978, 568), who recognize that "in most hospitals, a rich albeit esoteric folklore flourishes providing a much needed outlet for doctors and nurses who are under almost continual round-the-clock pressure." They examine the term *gomer*, a word used to describe older, difficult, usually alcoholic patients at Veterans Administration hospitals, concluding that the term strengthened in-group solidarity, provided an outlet for anxiety and frustration, and relieved stress. Similarly, David Paul Gordon (1983), sociologist Howard S. Becker (1993), and folklorist Stephen D. Winick (2004) independently argue that folk speech targets difficult patients that demand unwarranted or unneeded attention and so expresses frustration and release hostility. Folklorist Kathleen Odean (1995) examines a range of "anal folklore" in medicine, concluding that it expressed hostility toward patients and medical professionals, produced feelings of superiority, released tension, expressed the breaking of taboos, and provided group cohesion. Physician Adam T. Fox and colleagues (2003) analyzes slang in British hospitals, noting that medical slang increased feelings of belonging and helped physicians cope with stress.[7] Anthropologist Anne Burson-Tolpin (1989, 1990) documents the playful speech registers of pediatricians arguing persuasively that such speech countered the instrumentality and rationality of biomedicine. Most of these authors concluded that such folklore reinforced group boundaries and strengthened in-group identity. These psychological and sociological functions are important and in many cases accomplished simultaneously, as humor is a multifunctional phenomenon. I do not, however, substantively engage with these aspects because they already have been thoroughly documented.

Others have approached folklore and medicine through narrative. Folklorist Lynwood Montell's *Tales of Kentucky Doctors* (2008) is a notable collection of stories from generalists who worked in solo practice in Kentucky, and folklorist Timothy R. Tangherlini's *Talking Trauma* (1998) on storytelling among EMTs examines the storytelling performances of first responders, focusing on graphic narratives of the horror they encounter in their daily work. Utilizing a phenomenological and discourse-centered approach, folklorist Katharine Young (1997) conducted extensive ethnographic work at a university hospital, examining how personhood was constituted and managed through the overlap of body and talk as people were transformed into patients in various medical encounters.

Studies of humor and vernacular speech within the medical field itself tend to be practical, examining whether humor is helpful or useful (McCreaddie and Wiggins 2008; Penson et al. 2005; Sobel 2006); whether it is ethical (McCrary and Christensen 1993; Watson 2011; Donnelly 1986); whether it creates a negative atmosphere or adversely affects training (Wear et al. 2009); and whether its risks outweigh its benefits (Berger, Coulehan, and Belling 2004). All of these studies reveal values, insights, and beliefs about a topic that is important to most people: the modern health care system.

My project builds on previous studies of medical speech to illustrate how and why the backstage occupational folklore of physicians is carnivalesque. It is of course impossible to generalize about humor, how it functions, or why it exists among the tens of thousands of physicians who practice within such a large context as organized medicine. Humor also varies widely according to individual inclination: some doctors use humor while others do not. Further, the use of humor is context dependent, meaning that the immediate social context shapes the emergence, functions, and meanings of humor in specific situations (Oring 2008). The meanings of laughter also vary. As literary scholar Stefan Horlacher (2009, 20) writes, "*The* laughter does not exist; there are only endlessly proliferating forms of laughter" (italics mine). Laughter is a bodily eruption of the semiotic, so while laughter signifies, its meaning is somewhat inexpressible (Thomas 1997). Not all laughter, for example, is associated with humor. Laughter may be a response to humor, but it also may be strategic, or it may lie somewhere in between (A. Brock 2008). Laughter in medical contexts is no different. There is joyful laughter, surprised laughter, derisive laughter, and the laughter of exhaustion, to name a few. Carnivalesque laughter is ambivalent and, ideally, liberating. As literary scholar Renate Lachmann (1988–89, 134) explains, "The principle of [carnivalesque] laughter, which suspends this [cosmic] terror by translating it into the language of the material and the corporeal, a can thus be interpreted as *the* principle regenerating culture." In other words, carnivalesque laughter is laughter based on the body and functions as a form of renewal, so it is unsurprising it exists in medical contexts.

Medical humor and folklore are closely connected to the institutional, organizational, and cultural contexts in which physicians are trained and work. The primary institutional context here is that of the hospital, which addresses more acute and critical issues than physicians in private practice. Teaching hospitals are where medical students and residents usually are trained and come to grips with their chosen profession. I therefore have limited my project to physicians in twentieth- and twenty-first-century teaching hospitals, a period that coincides with the rise of institutionalized medicine. I have, however, also included historical examples of folk humor about medicine throughout the book as points of comparison. These historical examples fall outside the scope of my analysis, but they provide important context because they contain themes, orientations, and perspectives that parallel ones in modern-day medical humor used by doctors themselves. Ultimately, I believe they have direct affinities.

When I use the term *care providers*, I specifically mean MDs, although the ideas likely are applicable to other health care workers in modified ways. Nurses, for example, have their own occupational culture that both overlaps with and deviates from that of physicians. Biomedical culture also is not monolithic: there are significant cultural variations in medicine from place to place and institution to institution as well as significant differences among medical specialties within single institutions. Yet as I explain in chapter 1 on medical training, doctors usually attend medical school in one location, move (often across the country) to another institution for residency, and may move a third time if they pursue one or more fellowships. This enforced mobility creates a broad, occupationally grounded culture. As physician Dr. Brian Goldman (2014, 22) comments in his book of medical argot called *The Secret Language of Doctors*, it's "not about what goes on at Mount Sinai Hospital but rather about what goes on in hospitals across North America." In fact, many variations of the folklore I identify can also be found internationally in English-speaking countries such as England and Australia as well as countries where English is not predominant, such as Iran, Japan, and Brazil. Iranian emergency room doctors, for example, engage in a practice also found in the US in which physicians attempt to shunt patients off onto other doctors to lighten their heavy workloads (Mizrahi 1986). In the US, this is known as "buffing" and "turfing"—one "buffs" a patient to make them look "good" (meaning appropriate for transfer) in order to "turf" them, that is, move the patient to another service. The variation of this practice in Iran is a humorous reinterpretation of a basic medical check: from airway-breathing-circulation to airway-breathing-*circule*, where the term *circule* apparently refers to a purposefully false patient out-referral (to "refer out" means to refer a patient to someone else) (Mirhosseini and Fattahi 2010). Such occupational folklore arises in the specifics of Western medical training and the organization of work rather than identity features such as geographic location, ethnicity, or religion that often factor into the basis of culture.

The Medical Carnivalesque

As noted previously, the term *carnivalesque* is borrowed from literary theorist Mikhail Bakhtin ([1968] 1984) who coined the term to characterize the comic writings of French Renaissance author François Rabelais (1494–1553). Rabelais's best-known work is *The Life of Gargantua and Pantagruel,* a five-volume series that depicts the life and times of two giants named Panurge and Pantagruel, the adventures of which are filled with a cacophony of images including thrashings, curses, sex, eating and drinking, war, feasts, and oaths. The works are entirely over the top. They were so controversial that the writings were condemned by church authorities and complex enough to have engaged scholars for centuries.

Bakhtin argues that Rabelais's work was steeped in a thousand-year-old culture of folk humor that culminated in the Middle Ages and found its way into the literary works of early modern authors such as Shakespeare, Cervantes, and Rabelais. According to Bakhtin ([1968] 1984, 5), this ancient culture of folk humor and the laughter that accompanied it, which he termed *carnivalesque,* existed outside the more official and serious aspects of medieval society (in particular the church) and was found in carnivals, ritual spectacles and marketplace festivals, comic verbal compositions, and the free and familiar common speech of the people in the marketplace.

The concept of the carnivalesque ordinarily is found in festival studies, where it generally is understood as a potentially transgressive, temporary liberation from social norms, usually during times of celebration and accompanied by laughter and forms of play (e.g. Santino 2017; Gabbert 2011, 2019). Common examples include pre-Lenten festivals, such as Mardi Gras in the United States and Carnival celebrations in Europe and Latin America. People use feasting, drink, costume, alcohol, sleep-deprivation, and other forms of play to create a "time out of time" (Falassi 1987) in which received truths are questioned, parodied, or inverted; social statuses are rearranged or transgressed; and society is temporarily transformed.

"Carnival," as described by Bakhtin, not only existed in actual pre-Lenten festivities but also as a framework of communication in which people interacted and spoke freely with each other without regard for status or hierarchies. Ordinary rules of etiquette and norms of politeness were overlooked; established norms, social restrictions, and rules of society did not apply; and received truths were deemed relative and temporary rather than eternal and determined. The laughter associated with this framework of communication hinged on travesty, transgression, and parody, presenting false, absurd or distorted representations of official ideology and culture. Yet the purpose of carnival laughter was not derisive mockery or moral condemnation (Bakhtin [1968] 1984, 62). It was an ambivalent, collective laughter with a philosophical bent, a primary way to defeat fear. Carnival and carnival laughter created new meanings by offering alternate, comedic ways of looking at the world, a temporary liberation from existing power relations and normative social structures.

The medical carnivalesque draws on Bakhtin's ideas and proposes that a similar framework of communication exists in modern organized medicine. The medical carnivalesque entails a nexus of humor, play, playful speech, travesty, and laughter. It questions, inverts, or overturns established medical truths and ideals and in doing so provides a temporary alternative to existing medical norms. The term *peek and shriek*, for example, is sometimes used by surgeons. It refers to an unhappy surgical situation in which a patient is brought into the operating room, the abdomen is opened up, the surgeon realizes that the patient has a problem that cannot be fixed (such as widespread, inoperable cancer), and the abdomen is closed again (Goldman 2014, 290). This is a horrible, tragic situation (sometimes called a "horrendoma" [Burson-Tolpin 1990], a parodic, slang term for a terrible medical condition) for both patient and surgeon. It is terrible news for the patient since the patient likely will die, and it is bad for the surgeon because they can't do anything. Phrases such as *peek and shriek* emerge in large, bureaucratic institutions such as teaching hospitals and target some of the most serious and official issues with which medicine routinely engages, including death, disease, the body, and technocratic expertise. These phrases transgress official medical norms through inversion, playfulness, and parody by presenting those norms in a new, comic light. In this example, the phrase overturns normative ideas that surgeons are powerful and capable (e.g., "heroes"); that they are imperturbable; and that medical expertise will save the patient. As Dr. Marcus Burnstein reflects, "I think *peek and shriek* is a quick way of getting the message across that you encountered a disaster and *found yourself to be useless* [italics mine]" (quoted in Goldman 2014, 291). Such speech turns the biomedical world upside down by revealing it as fragile and contingent rather than authoritative and powerful. This example also contests conventional scholarly characterizations of medicine as hierarchical, reductive, normative, and rationalized (see Lupton 2003) through its emphasis on an emotional rather than technocratic response.

That said, however, a carnival mode in organized medicine is not a radical, permanent transformation of medical hierarchies and values, nor is it even particularly progressive. Like other deeply rooted institutions—such as the medieval Catholic Church, modern state governments, or the university system—organized medicine is powerful, conservative, and patriarchal. It is slow to change, and deep-seated change is difficult to enact. The carnivalesque seems progressive because it challenges normative ideals and offers alternatives to existing presumptions, but scholars have recognized that the reversals, mockery, and inversions of carnival mostly reinforce dominant cultural ideals (Russo 1986; Ware 2007; Stukator 2001). According to the widely accepted "safety-valve" theory, for example, pre-Lenten Carnival allowed the masses to blow off steam against the elites, thereby avoiding actual change and possible revolution. Carnival was *licensed* excess and transgression, a period of temporary liberation from social norms that was sanctioned by officials and so ultimately reinforced existing power structures. Carnival intimates change and provides visions of alternate realities, for example in areas of gender (N. Davis 1978). Those realities, however, are rarely achieved permanently. Renate Lachmann (1988–89, 125) observes that "the provocative, mirthful inversion of prevailing institutions . . . offers a permanent alternative to official culture—even if it ultimately leaves everything as it was before," while human geographers Neil Ravenscroft and Paul Gilchrist (2009, 37) note, "Carnival did not challenge the presence or power of Church or state but upheld the political order, despite the fact that such revelry might foster a utopian radicalism." They also point out that even carnivalesque transgressions have limits, as there are still norms that govern codes of conduct (Ravenscroft and Gilchrist 2009).

One reason carnivalesque transgressions reinforce hierarchies is that they rely on preexisting categories and ideas as the basis on which hilarity is posited, thus reproducing existing power structures. The frameworks themselves are not challenged. This certainly is the case in medicine, where a carnivalesque orientation does not seriously challenge patriarchal power structures but usually reinforces those structures, often by noting where transgressions lie and exaggerating them for comic purposes. In the previously given example, *peek and shriek* acknowledges the fallibility and occasional uselessness of surgeons. At the same time, it reinforces the idea that surgeons are ordinarily competent and take care of the patient's problem. The phrase does not interrogate frameworks of presumptions about surgeons, preexisting ideas about doctors as heroes, or the category of "surgeon" itself. The carnivalesque in medicine offers temporary alternatives to existing norms, not permanent change.

Another important aspect of the medical carnivalesque is its relation to suffering. In Bakhtin's formulation, carnival laughter defeats cosmic terror by transforming it into what Bakhtin ([1968] 1984, 91) calls a gay and festive monster. In medical contexts carnival laughter is less about cosmic terror than about suffering.[8] Medicine seeks to alleviate human suffering but frames suffering according to a clinical perspective, meaning that it treats suffering as a problem to be solved in patients. This perspective overlooks the fact that suffering is a *cultural* element in medicine. Patients suffer, but care providers can also suffer because suffering is an intersubjectively constituted phenomenon (Kleinman and Kleinman 1991). Care providers relieve the suffering of others, and this task can cause them to suffer as well. Even the phrase *peek and shriek* points to the suffering of the doctor since the inoperable situation causes the surgeon to shriek in horror. Further, the work physicians do with patients places them continuously outside of social and cultural norms because medical work on the body often breaches social and cultural boundaries. Physicians can be said to be in a position of permanent liminality and ambivalence, and this position arguably produces suffering in the physician. Finally, the physician role means that the care provider consistently puts the patient (that is, "work") above their own needs. Coupled with an occasionally toxic work culture that emphasizes perfectionism, grueling work hours and toughness, and engenders shame about needing help (Symon 2018), a situation emerges in which care providers may suffer alongside their patients. Unfortunately, the suffering of care providers is rarely acknowledged or addressed in the scholarly literature. Some activists even argue that there is a purposeful silencing by the medical community on this issue (Symon 2018). These conditions create an institutionalized context in which suffering is always present or lingers in the shadows.

There are several reasons why a carnivalesque orientation exists in modern organized medicine. First, carnivalesque orientations challenge institutional power. Carnival fully developed in the medieval period in Europe in opposition to the dominant institutional power of the Catholic Church. There are few institutions in the modern world that wield power in the same way as the medieval church, but organized medicine as it exists in teaching hospitals is formidable. The teaching hospital is what Erving Goffman (1961) calls a "total institution" or an "instrumental formal organization," terms that come from his midcentury work on psychiatric hospitals. Examples of total institutions include hospitals, prisons, schools, monasteries, and the various branches of the military. Such institutions have (or at least seem to have) near-total control over their "inmates"[9] or residents, and they are characterized by inspections, hierarchies, divisions between staff and inmates/residents, discipline, obedience tests, admission procedures, barriers to the wider world, dispossession of property, and the collection of detailed, personal information.[10] Patients in health care facilities, for example, receive an expert diagnosis; undergo surveillance in the form of health monitoring and checkups; and, as Goffman observes, endure obedience tests that are framed by medical language as "compliance." Goffman (1961, 6) writes that "various enforced activities are brought together into a single rational plan purportedly designed to fulfill the official aims of the institution," whether that aim be to heal the sick (in the case of hospitals),[11] reform the criminally minded (in the case of jails and prisons), maintain a sacred lifestyle (in the case of monasteries), or some other purpose.[12]

Total institutions generate alternative frameworks of communication due to their inherently unequal power dynamics. Goffman (1961, 171–320) writes about the existence of an "underlife of the public institution," and folklorists have documented antithetical modes of communication in institutions such as summer camps (Mechling 2019), although they don't identify them as carnivalesque. In teaching hospitals, this alternative mode of communication exists among staff rather than patients and includes not only doctors but also nurses, physician's assistants, and other care providers. Business scholars Robert I. Westwood and Allanah Johnson (2013, 221) write that in organizations, humor "can also express resistance to and subvert the dominant social order, reveal and play with the paradoxes, irrationalities and incongruities of modern organizational life, and expose a counterpoint to organizational and managerial absurdities." A carnivalesque orientation acts as a centrifugal force, promoting openness and ambivalence against the institution's centripetal impulses, which push toward closed and standardized systems (Lachmann 1988–89, 116).

It could be argued that a truly authentic carnivalesque atmosphere at a hospital would entail patients taking over the hospital and acting as doctors and nurses, since patients are the ones who lack power and the carnivalesque entails power reversals. This is accurate and would be one radical form. Patients, however, are not really part of the broader occupational culture of medicine. Patients are the object of care and attention, and they structure the way in which hospital work is organized; however, patients are not insiders to hospital culture, and they do not have a folk hospital culture because they stay there temporarily (Mechling 2019). The care providers who work in medical institutions are the core of medical culture, and it is their lives that are regulated by the institution to a much larger extent. As one medical proverbial saying goes, patients eventually leave the hospital one way or another, but the staff are always there. Physicians have a unique position within this occupational context. On the one hand, they hold power, and it is by virtue of their status that they participate in a carnivalesque orientation that targets the institution. On the other hand, physician power is circumscribed and institutionally regulated by innumerable factors, including administrative protocols, federal and state laws, insurance regulations, and technology. As Jay Mechling (2019, 669) observes: "In truth, the staff often experiences the same lack of agency [as the residents] in the total institution." The medical carnivalesque emerges in contradistinction to the institution by those who work there.

Second, a carnivalesque perspective emerges in medicine because the carnivalesque challenges institutionalized, authoritative truths. Bakhtin ([1968] 1984, 4) describes the pervasive medieval culture of folk carnival humor as "a boundless world of humorous forms and manifestations [that] opposed the official and serious tone of medieval ecclesiastical and feudal culture," and later explains that "one might say that carnival celebrated temporary liberation from the prevailing truth and from the established order" (10). Medicine—and its close relation, science—is one of the most authoritative discourses that has emerged since the Enlightenment. Particularly throughout the twentieth century and into the twenty-first, medicine and science have determined what counts as knowledge and truth, what is viable, and, to a broad extent, what is reality.[13] The knowledge/truths they produce have come to structure the reality of ordinary people's lives. Evidence-based medicine, for example, relies on scientific findings to determine practice, and medical recommendations inform laws and regulations that govern the lives of millions of people because they are perceived to be accurate. Medicine also determines what counts as normal and what counts as deviant and, therefore, potentially immoral (Foucault 1973). Further, the official speech register of medicine is largely formal and technocratic, what Richard Bauman (following Bakhtin) calls "authoritative speech," which is speech that does not allow for multiple perspectives but rather situates itself as a single purveyor of truth.

Rabelais connected medicine directly to carnival through the language of the marketplace, specifically among the cries of sellers, circus barkers, and vendors of medicinal cures. Medicine in the Middle Ages consisted not only of academic medical knowledge but also the theatrics and advertising by mountebanks and quacks in public arenas. Bakhtin included such medical theatrics in his analysis. Today most physicians no longer actively hawk drugs, and the aspects of medical showmanship have been taken over by medical television advertising.[14] However, nicknames and slang terms for various specialties, such as labeling anesthesiologists "gas passers," are a modern way physicians humorously undermine medicine as authoritative truth, a comic vein explored in chapter 5. Medical specialties represent highly technical training, but among doctors, urologists might be known as "pecker checkers" or "plumbers," surgeons as "cowboys," internists as "fleas," and orthopedists as "carpenters." As C. Peterson (1998, 673) remarks, "Medical slang *creates new meanings in the relationship of physicians . . . to their own acquisition of clinical knowledge and expertise* and above all to the health care system itself" (italics mine). Such terms degrade and debase medical expertise, although again they ultimately uphold the status quo of expert knowledge since they are used only by peers and their comic efficacy depends on equal relations of power among participants. Physicians are instruments of expert knowledge, and they use humor and laughter to temporarily overturn, question, and parody the institutionalized knowledge/ truth that they embody.

Third, a carnivalesque mode emerges in medicine because medicine focuses on the body, and a focus on the body was the primary concern of old manifestations of the carnivalesque. In the medieval and early modern periods, carnival[15] conjured depictions of what Bakhtin calls the "grotesque body," which were representations of the human body as large, exaggerated, cosmic, universal, and hyperbolic. As I explain in chapter 4, the term *grotesque* does not mean "gross" but rather is a fundamental aspect of "grotesque realism," which is the aesthetic style associated with carnival frameworks. The grotesque body includes exaggerated orifices such as mouths and noses and ears as well as associations with the lower torso, such as the belly and intestines, the anus, and the genitals, or what Bakhtin refers to as the "bodily lower material stratum." These images are complex, but they constitute a metaphorical conception of a "becoming" body that references life through actions such as eating, digestion, elimination, reproduction and birth, and death through images of disease and dismemberment, including anatomization for carnivalesque purposes.

Rabelais was a physician and influenced by ancient medical ideas, such as humoral theory. These ancient theories informed Rabelais's concept of the grotesque body. The grotesque body, for example, is not an individual body; it is collective, cosmic, and reflects the known universe (see Bakhtin [1968] 1984, 354–58). The grotesque body is also transgressive, presumably contrasting with the idealized perfection of the restored body of Christ; it, therefore, resisted institutionalized religious power.

The body continues affiliations with collectivity in the modern world. It is understood less as cosmic and universal than as a stand-in for various orders of social organization such as the nation-state or the family. Conceptualized thus, operations on the body are always operations on culturally constructed categories, and so the body is an important site for the application of power. This is particularly true in medicine, which seeks to produce normative, idealized medical bodies (white, masculine, young, healthy, and able-bodied) by attempting to control and contain biological processes. In doing so medicine produces and reproduces cultural categories of domination and marginality, including categories of gender and deviancy. It is not surprising then that carnivalesque images of the grotesque body emerge. It is a useful foil to the idealized medical body, reflecting both the realities of the patient bodies with which physicians work and offering a stark contrast to heteronormative ideals.

Morbid obesity, for example, is associated with imagery of the grotesque body. Research on fatness reveals that morbidly obese bodies are considered transgressive and that they are indicators of the carnivalesque because of their large size and the exaggerated protuberance of the belly (or pannus). Morbidly obese patients present physicians with unique challenges, leading physicians to joke or speak about obesity in coded ways. In Indiana, for example, a state known in the early 2000s for obesity, obese patients might be colloquially measured in "Hoosier units." A single Hoosier unit was 220 pounds (100 kilograms), so a person who weighed two Hoosier units weighed about 440 pounds. This informal weight measurement system is not limited to Indiana but can be found throughout the Midwest, including Illinois, Wisconsin, Iowa, and Minnesota as a Chicago unit, a Wisconsin unit, or a Minnesota unit; at Case Western Reserve in Ohio, patients were measured in "clinic units" (Goldman 2014, 193–94), again illustrating that medical culture is occupationally based.

Such talk reinforces normative medical ideals by noting where bodily transgressions exist. Like sexist mnemonics, it may be shocking to outside audiences. Most physicians don't engage in this talk at all, and those who do only do so in close company. Abusive speech based on the body, however, is part of a carnivalesque framework and in Terry Eagleton's (2019a, 35) words, carnival can be "violent and vituperative."[16] Not all carnivalesque aspects are humorous but instead may be callous, insensitive, or cruel. Abusive speech is not funny but ambivalent, and it is associated with the grotesque body, which is a body that literally cannot be contained. Such images challenge the idealized, normative, and medicalized body while at the same time functioning as a form of social control by acknowledging the existence of an opposite.

A final reason that a carnivalesque framework emerges in organized medicine is that Rabelais's carnivalesque already had strong medical elements. As a physician and an anatomist, Rabelais wrote serious medical treatises and performed a public dissection in 1537 (Bakhtin [1968] 1984, 159). Medical references emerge in his humorous writings as a core component. He included parodic, exaggerated, and nonsensical references to various diseases, cures, drugs, and descriptions of the body throughout his comic writings. Bakhtin points out that medical aspects are essential to Rabelais's writings, although he does not develop the idea: "Images of the physician and the medical element are organically linked in the novel [that is, in Rabelais's works] with the entire traditional system [carnival] of images" (360).

Bakhtin observes that Rabelais's carnivalesque was based in popular folk humor, and popular folk humor often targeted medicine. Jokes and tales found in the "Facetiae" collection of Poggio Bracciolini (d. 1459) are one example of the broad comic folk tradition on which Rabelais drew.[17] Bracciolini was born near Florence in 1380 and a collection of his humorous tales was published in Latin in 1470 in two volumes. The volumes contain jests concerning women, priests, and physicians, among other people. Tale 87, "A quack who attended asses" (Bracciolini 1879, 139), for example, is about a man who knows nothing about medicine but decides to practice it by simply putting things in pills. The quack is celebrated as a learned physician despite his lack of medical knowledge when his pills supposedly help a peasant find his animal. Tale 109, "A Sly Physician," (173) is about an "ignorant but sly, physician" who teaches his student to diagnose patients by looking around the room to see what they have eaten and then blaming the illness on gluttony. The student eventually leaves to practice medicine on his own. He enters the room of a patient, sees the saddle of an ass, and accuses his patient of having eaten the ass. The student is ridiculed and humiliated for his absurd diagnosis. Another tale, 61, is about a woman who is sick and calls in a doctor (178). The physician, who is described in the tale as "ignorant," asks to see her urine. The urine is accidentally switched with that of a young female servant and the doctor, upon inspecting it, declares that the cure for the woman's sickness is sexual intercourse. The patient's husband has intercourse with her, she is cured, and the doctor's "prescription" is hailed as a success.

Bracciolini's jokes poke fun at gullibility, at commoners who pretend to be something they are not, and at physicians. Certainly there were respectable physicians during Bracciolini's era, but such jokes intimated that physicians might also be sly and ignorant. They suggest that medicine may be successfully practiced by common fools and quacks who are interested in sex and money. Similar ideas about medicine permeate Rabelais's writings, including references to gluttony, urine, fake prescriptions, quackery, and sexual intercourse. By the early modern period, these themes were familiar enough to have solidified into a stock physician character in theatrical performances of *commedia dell'arte*. This stock character was a buffoon, defined as a carnival figure characterized by his "belly" and not his intellect (Rudlin 1994, 101).

Research Approaches

My interest in the backstage occupational and humorous folklore of medicine is long-standing, but it arose largely circumstantially because my spouse went to medical school. I do not come from a medical family. Like most other people, I had little idea what the implications were when he made that decision. As a spouse, I had glimpses into the education and training of doctors as he made his way through medical school, a residency in internal medicine, and a fellowship in pulmonary/critical care. I discovered that doctoring is both gratifying and relentless, transforming those who undertake it and those around them. Medical training profoundly impacted my family and personal life in ways that are difficult for nonmedical people to understand. The arguments I make in this book about suffering as an unacknowledged part of medical culture directly stem from this impact, as family issues of mental illness and addiction were exacerbated by an occupational culture that discourages physicians from seeking help and frames provider health issues as weakness. These circumstances compelled me to reframe my original project, which I initially conceptualized as one on humor and death, to a broader examination of suffering and the carnivalesque.

This is not an ethnographic project in the conventional sense, and I do not consider it as such. I am part of a medical family but not an insider to medicine. Researchers historically have immersed themselves in the field to produce ethnographies, often training or even living alongside their research partners to gain understanding in a method known as participant observation. The classic example of participant observation in medicine is Howard S. Becker and colleagues' study of medical school titled *Boys in White* (1961). In the age of transnational flows and digital communication networks, notions of what constitutes "the field" have been thoroughly dismantled, but I did not attend medical school, engage in medical training, or shadow physicians in hospitals for months on end. Such an approach was impractical given my work and life constraints as a faculty member, mother, and marriage partner. Instead, my main method of information-gathering has been ongoing informal discussions with friends who are physicians, their spouses, and physician acquaintances, conversations that have been invaluable in the formation of the ideas here.

I conducted a more limited form of observation by occasionally shadowing physicians, including preliminary research by observing shock-trauma rounds in 2006 at LDS Hospital in Salt Lake City and spending two days in the operating room in 2016 at the University of Utah hospital. These experiences helped me better understand generally what a day in the life of a doctor might look like. For examples of humorous content, I relied on published sources, informal conversations, the mass media, social media, and the internet. I also used books of humorous collectanea written by physicians; novels by physicians; and the work of medical sociologists and folklorists. Websites such as

GomerBlog, where physicians create content for other physicians, were quite valuable, including the user comments. I conducted more formal oral history interviews with physicians as an Archie Green Fellow (2019–20) for the Occupational Folklife Project at the Library of Congress American Folklife Center. Audio files, transcripts, and photographs are deposited at the American Folklife Center for those who are interested, and these materials constitute the first national collection of physician interviews (Gabbert 2019–2020). These formal interviews were less useful regarding humorous occupational folklore than my informal conversations and published sources. Talking about humor in formal interview settings usually made the humor unfunny for lack of appropriate social context, or interviewees were unable to think of examples for the same reason. The interviews instead provided extensive information about medical work and training, and many physicians talked openly about the role of suffering in their work, providing a physician-oriented perspective on their workaday lives.

These approaches mean that I do not address the immediate performance situation. Backstage occupational folklore emerges in socially situated interactions that are largely impossible to document firsthand. The actual situation in which a humorous utterance is made can be documented only after the fact (stand-up comedy is a notable exception, see Brodie 2014), which makes an analysis of the performance quite tricky. Instead of attempting to re-create performance situations, my analysis focuses on larger cultural and institutional contexts.

Examining playful backstage talk also brings ethical issues to the fore because of the topics it addresses. Play, playful speech, and laughter emerge in socially situated contexts and when taken out of those contexts can be radically misunderstood or misinterpreted. The audience for this humor is other doctors; it is very likely to be interpreted differently or misunderstood by anyone not a member of that group (Smith 2009). Some scholars have even suggested that medical humor should be off-limits to scholarly research because it is too controversial. Lawyers, for example, have suggested that physician humor might constitute medical malpractice (Schweikart 2020). Physicians themselves warn that medical humor is dangerous, evidenced by the comic disclaimer found on various websites, including a Facebook page for general surgery discussions and health-related blogs: "This post is for entertainment purposes only and likely contains humor only understood by those in a healthcare profession. Read at your own risk."

Physicians also are professionals who naturally are concerned about their reputations. No one wants to look bad because they joked among colleagues in a socially situated context that was likely stressful. I have only gratitude and utmost respect for the physicians who shared their experiences and viewpoints with me: everyone was incredibly insightful, thoughtful, and honest about their work. To help ensure their protection, I have given them pseudonyms and removed identifying factors such as location of work. In most cases where I used a direct quotation or story from an interview, I returned portions of the unpublished manuscript to the physicians I quoted and requested separate permission to use that quotation or statement so participants could see how the quotation was being used within the context of the book. I hope that these practices suffice to offset potential ethical dilemmas.[18]

Finally, doctoring remains a profession of white privilege, as the section on medical student demographics in chapter 1 illustrates. Organized medicine also is a domain of racism, classism, and a good deal of sexism. This book does not directly dismantle the racist, classist, and patriarchal underpinnings of organized medicine: that work has been done by others who focus on vernacular, ethnic, or lay medical perspectives. My project outlines the carnivalesque tradition within medicine, a tradition that ultimately is grounded in and likely perpetuates the racist, classist, and white privileged perspectives that permeate organized medicine in general, despite its seemingly oppositional stance to institutionalized directives.

It is also true that physicians and other upper-middle-class groups have been protected from the documentation, classification, and analysis that accompanies research. This is in part due to the discipline of folklore's desire to document the perspectives of underrepresented populations and in part due to lack of access. My access is the direct result of my own privilege. As both a white professor at an academic research institution and the spouse of a physician, my position gave me access to doctors, legitimizing me as a valid researcher and someone who could be trusted. For example, it would have been very difficult to schedule interviews if I had not had physicians' private cell phone numbers and a sabbatical, which gave me a large amount of unstructured time to pursue this work. Surgeons in particular could not tell me their schedule in advance, and mostly texted the morning of the day when they had an hour or two available. I had to be available when they had time. I hope that I have used this privilege well by furthering others' understanding of medicine as a cultural institution and of the culture of doctors as an occupational group.

Chapter Summaries

The argument of this book is twofold. First, it argues that suffering is an unrecognized cultural component of the practice of medicine. Second, it argues

that the specific comic vein characterizing much medical humor is the carnivalesque, an ancient orientation in which themes of life, death, and the body are
central. These two aspects, suffering and carnival, are interconnected. Chapter
1, "'Like Drinking from a Firehose': The Organization of Medical Education,
Training, and Work," provides an overview of the length and nature of physician training, an intense period that instills core medical values of hard work,
self-sacrifice, perfectionism, and lack of self-care in trainees. The chapter includes stories of getting into medical school and what medical school is like, as
well as information on postgraduate training such as residency and fellowship.
It also details testing and licensing procedures and includes statistical and demographic information about who becomes a doctor in the US. Women have
made large inroads into medicine since the turn of the twenty-first century
and have affected the cultural milieu; however, underrepresented racial and
ethnic groups remain disproportionally small, and most doctors, male and
female, come from financially stable families. This chapter also covers some
ritual aspects of becoming a physician, such as the white coat ceremony and
match day. Because the medical carnivalesque is an occupational phenomenon,
this chapter provides important background.

Chapter 2, "'Living the Dream': Suffering, Moral Injury, and Trauma in
Medical Practice" argues that suffering permeates medical work and is an important cultural aspect of medicine. Physicians and other health care workers
may suffer because of their work, yet this suffering is hidden due to the occupational focus on patients. Specifically, physicians witness the suffering of their
patients. It also is their job to relieve suffering as part of their work. Failure to do
so can cause suffering. Finally, their highly competitive work environment can
exacerbate suffering because of the lack of institutionalized support. Suffering
constitutes the "deep context" for the medical humor described in the rest of
the book and the broader concept of the medical carnivalesque. The chapter
includes statistics about physician suicide rates, examples from the COVID-19
pandemic, and excerpts from interviews on the topic of physician suffering.

Chapter 3 is titled "Death, Life, and Other Absurdities." One important
manifestation of the carnivalesque is the mediation of life and death. This is
also the basis of doctoring. This chapter focuses on death-related folklore in
medicine, contextualizing it within the broader Western denial of death that
has occurred over the past 160 years in which people rarely, if ever, see dead
bodies. I argue that much death-related folklore targets biomedical responses
to death and disease, which tend toward rationalization, technocracy, and
control. The first part of the chapter explores humor and folklore in the gross
anatomy lab. The second part of the chapter explores slang and colloquial

terms for death, the dead, and the dying that circulate among some medical personnel.

Chapter 4, "Bodies of Humor: The Medicalized and the Grotesque," examines speech about patient bodies.[19] Physicians tell stories about the strange things patient bodies do (or have been done to them), and they tell jokes and personal experience narratives about the ways in which bodies transgress boundaries. I argue that the contrasting images of the controlled, medicalized body and the transgressive, grotesque body underlie this folkloric corpus of stories about feces and other pollutants; gigantism and comments about fatness; and narratives about disease and dismemberment.

Chapter 5, "'I Can Fix It': Spurious and Expert Knowledge," explores the ways in which medical knowledge as an authoritative truth is undermined in intragroup folklore about medical specialties and in beliefs about luck. This chapter focuses on humor that targets the knowledge of specialties like orthopedics, anesthesiology, psychiatry, and surgery, arguing that this folklore fits within the larger framework of the carnivalesque, which historically embraces charlatanism and mountebanks and suggests that physicianship and showmanship are interconnected.

In the conclusion, I speculate on the relations between suffering and carnival vis-à-vis the concept of transcendence and advocate for the nation to move toward a more humane health care system.

Notes

1. I am grateful to Mark Damen, professor of history and classics at Utah State University, for this helpful reference.

2. For an excellent history of the idea of "humor" as it separated over time from physiology and in relation to the development of the idea of the individual, see Wickberg 1998.

3. Folklorist Alan Dundes and Thomas Hauschild (1983) document aggressive antisemitic jokes told by Holocaust aggressors, arguing that, while awful, they at least acknowledge the horrors of the Holocaust.

4. The terms used to describe this type of humor draw on the biases inherent in colorism, which characterize problematic, unhealthy, aggressive, or unpleasant aspects of culture as "dark" or "black."

5. Throughout the book, I use the title "Dr." to refer to physicians and not to PhDs to avoid confusion.

6. As definitions of folklore and folklife expanded during the 1960s and 1970s (McCarl 1978), studies of white-collar professions emerged in addition to those

of the working classes, including those that observed trial lawyers (Schrager 1999), physician-patient interactions (Dundes and Pagter 1975), employees of various institutions (Jones 1994; Christensen 1988), and the iconic occupations of particular regions such as New York (Groce 2010), in particular an excellent in-depth ethnography of Wall Street (Ho 2009). Despite this work, however, it remains true that upper-middle-class professions are the province of sociologists rather than folklorists, an ongoing orientation that prompted anthropologist Charles Briggs (2012) to encourage folklorists to "study up" in health care, meaning to include more powerful and privileged stakeholders as subjects rather than limiting studies to the disenfranchised, a focus that some scholars have argued perpetuates racism (see Prahlad 2021).

7. Folklorists Lauren Dundes, Michael B. Streiff, and Alan Dundes (1999) also examined the medical proverbial expression "when you hear hoofbeats, think horses, not zebras," a saying that advises doctors first to look for the more common causes of disease rather than the rare ones. For additional studies, see Trahant 1981, Moore 1991, Grayson 1981.

8. Humor studies have established that humor often functions as a source of relief. Carnival laughter in medicine relieves suffering, but here my point is that the medical carnivalesque is grounded in a pervasive context of suffering and less on its functional components.

9. In using the term *inmate*, Goffman (1961, 13) literally means a person "on the inside," and so the term applies to any resident of a total institution, not just people who are jailed, which is the more common sense of the term. *Resident* today is a more commonly used term.

10. Hospitals of the past, however, were likely not as bleak as Goffman described them; some critics have noted that Goffman overlooked humanistic aspects of 1950s mental hospitals, which at the time were experimenting with therapies such as dance and art (Gambino 2013; Bengtsson and Bülow 2016). Goffman himself acknowledged that his description of total institutions was an idealization. He stated that total institutions varied in nature from one to another and that no actual institution fully possessed all of his described characteristics.

11. More accurately, one physician wryly noted that the main purpose of hospitals is to discharge patients and make sure they don't come back for at least thirty days.

12. Philosopher and historian Michel Foucault outlines similar practices in his 1975 book *Discipline and Punish*, which traces the emergence of the modern penal form as it emerged at the end of the eighteenth century. Foucault argues that society (specifically, France) developed a science of discipline in this time period, which was a new way of wielding power that could be found in schools, hospitals, the military, prisons, and other organizations. This science of discipline involved similar activities to those Goffman describes, such as extreme

regimentation, timed control of activities, hierarchies, and judgments made by specialists. See chapter 4 for more discussion of the body in relation to this new science of discipline.

13. Since the rise of the internet, however, scientific inquiry as a valid source of knowledge has come under attack, illustrating that these discourses are not as authoritative as they once were. One recent example is the debate about the nature and cause of climate change, despite an overwhelming amount of scientific evidence that climate change is caused by humans. Another example are arguments against proven methods of eliminating the transmission of viruses, such as the wearing of masks and vaccination during the COVID-19 pandemic. For an analysis of physician folkloric responses to these challenges, see Gabbert 2023.

14. I am grateful to my colleague Jeannie Thomas for this suggestion.

15. Throughout this book I have capitalized the word *Carnival* when I refer to an actual pre-Lenten celebration and use the lower-case form *carnival* to refer to a generalized atmosphere or mode of communication.

16. Renate Lachmann (1988–89, 122) writes about cases in which inversion led to the establishment of new political orders that were horrifying. Apparently Ivan the Terrible usurped carnival inversion for his own ends, establishing a counterstate with its own laws to become a theater of cruelty.

17. I am very grateful to my colleague Christine Cooper-Rompato for pointing me to Bracciolini's *Facetiae* and for Cooper-Rompato's extensive feedback on the medieval materials found throughout the book.

18. Although participants agreed to have their interviews deposited at the American Folklife Center at the Library of Congress and made available to the public, I anonymized sources in this book to offer some degree of distance from the material.

19. My gratitude to Amber Cederström for the suggestion for this chapter title.

1

"Like Drinking from a Firehose"

The Organization of Medical Education, Training, and Work

Most people understand that being a doctor is difficult. Popular culture and the media play up stereotypes that physicians work long hours on very little sleep, often glamorizing the ethos of hard work and stoicism that prevails throughout the profession. But the details of how one actually becomes a doctor are less understood because the education and training of providers is lengthy and complicated. Physician training in the US combines formal academic training with the hands-on experiential learning associated more with traditional apprenticeships. In order to obtain a medical license, a person must minimally complete four years of medical school and at least one year of internship training. The reality, however, is that most doctors undergo a longer process: a three- to five-year residency, plus an additional one to three years (or more) of fellowship afterward, depending on the specialization. This prolonged timeline means that physicians are among the most specialized of white-collar professionals, with more requirements and a longer formal training period than lawyers, professors, or business leaders.

This chapter provides a general overview of how people become physicians, including the decision to become a doctor, the process of getting into medical school, and the postgraduate training that follows. It is not intended to be comprehensive but rather provide basic information. Readers wanting more detailed, experiential accounts should consult other sources. Many physicians enjoy medical school, and most appreciate the intense nature of medical training. But the way in which physician education, training, and work are organized also entails competitiveness, financial stress, a fear of failure, long hours, difficult work, strained personal relationships, a lack of proper food and sleep, and isolation from society. These elements, when combined with the difficult nature of medical work itself, contribute to an occupational ethos that teaches physicians consistently to deny their own needs in the context of work and so indirectly contribute to a culture of suffering. Understanding medical culture requires a grasp of physician education, training, and work and the environment in which such an ethos is cultivated.

Decision-Making: To Become a Doctor

Many physicians come from medical families. My spouse, for example, grew up in a medical family: his father was an orthopedic surgeon and his mother was a nurse, and he occasionally assisted his father in the operating room as a child. He was accustomed to the possibility of becoming a physician at a young age, although he was nearly thirty before he actually attended medical school. Dr. Brian Price, an orthopedic hand surgeon whom I interviewed in 2019, had a similar story: his father was a physician (a urologist named Dick), and Dr. Price also initially shied away from a career in medicine before entering medical school. Because medicine is partially an apprenticeship in which junior physicians are trained by more senior ones in a hands-on environment, it is unsurprising that the practice of medicine, like other occupations in which apprenticeships are important, may run in families. There often is an expectation in medical families that sons and daughters will go to medical school, although apparently more than a few balk before making the final decision.

For physicians who don't come from medical families, the decision to become a doctor takes a variety of forms. Dr. Susan Massey, a neonatologist and geneticist, for example, did not come from a medical family. As Dr. Massey explained, her grandmother wanted to be a doctor but never had the opportunity, so she pinned her hopes on her granddaughter. Dr. Massey said:

> She [my grandmother] would call me up every day—well, not every day, but when she talked she would ask me, "So, don't you want to be a doctor?" I'm like, "No, Grandma; I hate hospitals." And she would say, "I know; you're really good at math."
>
> And when I was in high school, she went into some nursing homes (after a stroke), and I spent a lot of time with the elderly in nursing homes. And she passed away my first year of college. . . . And that summer I was home, I was working, and my mother and I were driving to the beach one day, and it literally popped into my head, "I should be a doctor." And I always think I guess my grandma had more influence on the other side. [Laughs.] (Interview, November 5, 2019)

Dr. Mary Gibbs, a psychiatrist, was another example of a physician who did not come from a medical family. She originally was a music major in college and wanted to be a composer or a choir director. When it became clear that job prospects were scarce in those fields, she switched to her other love— science—and became a biology major with a chemistry minor. Eventually, she discovered medicine.

> **MG:** What changed my life was I was able to get a volunteer position at the Las Vegas medical examiner's office. And so, I started working there and I started—there's a term for what I did, it's a *diener* [laughs]—
>
> **LG:** A diener?
>
> **MG:** That's what they called them, yeah. Basically, an autopsy technician is the new, politically correct way to call it. So, I did autopsies. So, I removed the organs and gave them to the pathologist, and he would slice them and put them on slides. . . . So, then I thought, "Oh, maybe I should be a pathologist," you know? And so, I asked him, "How do I become what you do?" And he said, "Well you have to go to medical school." And I had no idea what that entailed, and I thought, "OK, well I guess I'll just go to medical school then." No big deal. Clearly, I was naive at the time. He talked about residencies and fellowships, and that went right over my head—I had no idea what he was talking about. I thought it was like a club, like a "fellow-ship" is like a club—like I didn't realize what that meant, in terms of training. So, I started researching how to get into medical school. And I did all the things, I checked all the boxes, I took all the classes I needed to take, I took the MCAT [Medical College Admission Test]. And I applied to medical school. And it was very tough. I didn't realize how hard it was to get into medical school. And I ended up going to the medical school in my state, which was actually the best decision, I think, because of the tuition (it was in-state tuition). And so my loans weren't quite as crazy.
>
> So, that's my getting into medical school story. (Interview, September 7, 2019)

Getting In

Medical school consists of four years of education after college/university. Students who successfully graduate from conventional allopathic medical schools are awarded the degree of MD (in Latin, *medicinae doctor*, or doctor of medicine), while those who attend an osteopathic medical school are awarded the degree of DO (doctor of osteopathic medicine).[1] The MD or DO degree is required for all physicians. These degrees constitute academic recognition only: they are not a medical license and do not allow graduates to legally practice.

Dr. Gibbs stated in the previous quotation that getting into medical school was tough. Acceptance is competitive, and spots are limited. Harvard Medical School admitted 226 students (a number that included 14 MD-PhD students) for the 2022 incoming class but received 6,914 applications for an admittance rate of approximately 3.3 percent (Harvard Medical School July 1, 2021–June 30, 2022).[2] Indiana University Medical School, a large, competitive midwestern school, enrolled 365 medical students for the incoming class of 2022 and received 6,805 applications for an admittance rate of approximately 5 percent (Indiana University School of Medicine 2022–2023).

Medical schools admit only the most highly qualified students, largely defined as students who have excellent grades in college science classes and strong MCAT scores. Such metrics are predictors of success in medical school, although not necessarily predictors of who will be a good doctor. Students entering medical school usually have completed a college or university education and obtained a bachelor's degree. Common premed majors include biology, chemistry, sociology, and statistics, but humanities degrees, particularly when combined with a second major in science, also are popular. Students in any major, however, can get into medical school as long as their grades are sufficiently high and they excel in their science classes, meaning that they are among the top students in the class. Successful applicants also score well on the MCAT, the required national standardized medical school entrance exam. According to the Princeton Review, a standardized entrance exam preparatory company, as of July 9, 2023, the average MCAT score for entering medical students in 2021–22 was between 511 and 512, with a score of 528 being the highest, while students' average grade point average was a 3.74. Many premed students also have completed significant service work, such as working with the poor or homeless, volunteering in hospitals, or working with refugees and other needy or underserved populations. People who are accepted into medical school then are highly motivated students who test well.

Applying to medical schools is expensive. The cost of taking the MCAT in 2023 was $330, and hopeful premed students also may pay additional money for tutors, practice exams, and extracurricular study materials in order to score well. Application fees for applying to medical schools vary but can be as high as $125 per application, and premed students may apply to as many as ten to fifteen schools. Such fees are only the beginning of the significant financial investment students make in their education. Medical school tuition is expensive and unlike college or university undergraduate education, there are few scholarships available. According to a spreadsheet provided by the Association of American Medical Colleges (AAMC), the average cost for tuition, fees, and insurance during the 2022–23 year for an in-state resident at a public medical school was $39,905 per year, and the average tuition for a nonresident was $63,780 per year. The cost of attending a private medical school for an in-state resident was $62,570 and for a nonresident was $64,103 (AAMC 2023). Tuition, however, even at such high rates, does not fully cover the institution's cost of educating a medical student and is partially subsidized; the remainder is paid through Medicare. Furthermore, these figures do not include the cost of room, board, textbooks, and other necessities, so the actual cost of attending medical school for students is higher. The University of Utah medical school website, for example, as of July 15, 2023, estimated the cost of books and supplies for the first year at $4,080. Most medical students pay for their school through federal loan programs and leave medical school with a substantial amount of debt, as it is nearly impossible to work an additional job while in school to pay for expenses. The amount of debt with which students graduate varies, but in 2019 the median debt was $200,000 (Budd 2020). This financial burden is compounded by the ongoing costs of professional licensing exams and board certifications (discussed in the sections below), which can affect students' decisions about which branches of medicine they enter and contribute to fear of and aversion to failure, since there are few alternative ways to pay back such heavy loans.

Medical students demographically come from higher socioeconomic backgrounds. Between the years 1988 and 2017, for example, somewhere between 73 and 79 percent of medical students came from the top two household income quintiles. For the decade of 2007–17, between 24 and 33 percent were in the top 5 percent of household income, while only 5 percent of students who matriculated during the same timeframe came from the lowest household income quintile (AAMC 2018). Further, the majority of medical students claim "white only" as their primary ethnic/racial category. An average of 9,818 self-identified white students matriculated each year between 2019–2023. As a point of comparison, students who identified as "Asian only" made up the second-largest racial/ethnic category with an average of about 5,057 students matriculating each year during that same period. Students who identified as "Black or African American only" matriculated at slightly under 1,843 total students per year, while "Hispanic, Latino, or of Spanish origin only" entered at an average of just over 1,488 students per year. "American Indian or Alaska Native Only" students matriculated at a rate of about 39 students per year, and there were 15.5

"Native Hawaiian or Other Pacific Islander Only" students who matriculated each year on average for the four-year period (AAMC 2022a).[3] Those figures generally hold true for graduates. From 2017 to 2022, the largest number of students who graduated identified as white, followed by students who identified as Asian, with students identifying as multiple race/ethnicity as the third-largest graduating group (AAMC 2022b).

Structural racism accounts for the ongoing lack of medical students from underrepresented groups. Nearly all medical schools excluded underrepresented groups until the 1960s, and so such students attended either Howard or Meharry medical schools. The AAMC pushed to increase the enrollment of students from underrepresented groups from the late 1960s through the 1980s, a move that was successful until the mid-1990s when a series of legal decisions in Texas and California excluded race, gender, and ethnicity from being included in admission criteria (Smedley, Butler, and Bristow 2004). This decision led to decreased numbers of applications from underrepresented groups and has remained so since. Additional structural barriers for underrepresented applicants identified by the Accreditation Council for Graduate Medical Education (ACGME) include educational disadvantages, a lack of mentorship, a lack of faculty of color at medical schools, poor or biased advising, low MCAT scores, and lack of access to physicians of color that lead to positive experiences (Smedley, Butler, and Bristow 2004). In 2009, the Liaison Committee of Medical Education required medical schools to develop programs designed to make medical education more accessible to diverse applicants as part of accreditation guidelines. These efforts resulted in an increase in the total number of diverse applications, but researchers at Penn State found that the proportion of applicants relative to overall shifting demographics statistically insignificant (Penn Medicine News 2019). Therefore, despite a more holistic approach to admissions and investment in pipeline programs, underrepresented applicants remain underrepresented.

Gender ratios are on par for men and women. Since at least the early 2000s, the number of women entering medical school has been only slightly lower than the number of men, and in recent years, the numbers have inverted so that women now constitute a slight majority. For the 2016–17 school year, for example, the number of matriculants in terms of gender was essentially the same (10,551 male, 50.2 percent, versus 10,474 female, 49.8 percent), while the 2017–18 year was the first time that female matriculants outnumbered men (10,516 male, 49.3 percent, versus 10,810 female, 50.7 percent). The ratio of female-to-male applicants continued to rise through the writing of this book: for the 2022–23 year, for example, there were 10,062 male matriculants (44.3 percent) and 12,630 female matriculants (55.6 percent) (AAMC 2022a). Yet while men and women enter medical school in approximately equal numbers, gender disparities become more obvious in later years as women gravitate toward specialties that offer more flexibility, such as dermatology and pediatrics, and less toward specialties like general surgery, pulmonology, and orthopedics, with the notable exception of obstetrics-gynecology.

Medical School

The exact nature of how medical school is organized varies from school to school and, to a certain degree, according to the interests of individual students. Many students are interested in clinical medicine and medical practice, meaning they envision themselves working with patients. Others may be more interested in research, and these interests inform the organization of their medical education. Typically, however, medical students spend their first two years taking basic science courses, including gross anatomy, biochemistry, pharmacology, microbiology, pathology, genetics, and cell biology, which usually are a mixture of classroom lectures and a significant amount of lab time. Many medical schools include additional curricular components such as classes or lectures on topics like ethics or the doctor-patient relationship, or schools may take an interdisciplinary approach that integrates relevant topics for shorter blocks of time. Some schools may also integrate clinical experience from the very beginning, meaning that students gain experience working with patients in hospitals or clinical settings as soon as they enter medical school. Students are identified as M1s, M2s, M3s, and M4s, indicating which year they are in medical school (an M1 is a first-year medical student). Students also begin paying malpractice insurance as an M1, which is included in the cost of tuition.

One of the most significant rites of passage for medical students is the well-known "white coat ceremony," which usually occurs at the beginning of medical school but may also occur at the end. During the ceremony, students don the white lab coat that symbolizes their physicianship for the first time, and they publicly take the Hippocratic oath (also known as a "pledge" rather than an oath), the medical oath of ethics that allegedly dates to ancient Greece and commonly is attributed to Hippocrates, the father of medicine.

There are many versions of the Hippocratic oath. It has been modified many times, and there is no standardized version required for all medical students. One common version is the "Declaration of Geneva," called so since it was drafted by the General Assembly of the World Medical Association in Geneva in 1948 (and has been modified a number of times since). It reads:

AS A MEMBER OF THE MEDICAL PROFESSION:
- I SOLEMNLY PLEDGE to dedicate my life to the service of humanity;
- THE HEALTH AND WELL-BEING OF MY PATIENT will be my first consideration;
- I WILL RESPECT the autonomy and dignity of my patient;
- I WILL MAINTAIN the utmost respect for human life;
- I WILL NOT PERMIT considerations of age, disease or disability, creed, ethnic origin, gender, nationality, political affiliation, race, sexual orientation, social standing or any other factor to intervene between my duty and my patient;
- I WILL RESPECT the secrets that are confided in me, even after the patient has died;
- I WILL PRACTICE my profession with conscience and dignity and in accordance with good medical practice;
- I WILL FOSTER the honor and noble traditions of the medical profession;
- I WILL GIVE to my teachers, colleagues, and students the respect and gratitude that is their due;
- I WILL SHARE my medical knowledge for the benefit of the patient and the advancement of healthcare;
- I WILL ATTEND TO my own health, well-being, and abilities in order to provide care of the highest standard;
- I WILL NOT USE my medical knowledge to violate human rights and civil liberties, even under threat;
- I MAKE THESE PROMISES solemnly, freely and upon my honor.[4]

The ritual donning of the white coat signals the students' transformation from layperson to student-physician, and it also is the first instance in which students are inducted into the professional hierarchies that will dominate their lives for the foreseeable future. In the past, in what might be termed "white coat folklore," the length of the white coat signaled one's status and position to others. The white coat itself meant that one was a physician, while the length and look of the white coat signified one's status. White coats for medical students and first-year interns were short, signaling their inferior position. Today, however, many different kinds of health providers may wear white coats, while doctors may or may not wear them at all.[5]

Students spend much of their time during the first two years studying and taking exams. The experience of the first two years commonly is described as trying to "drink from a firehose," meaning that the amount of information presented is torrential and that it is impossible to learn it all. Psychiatrist Dr. Susie Conrad described it as "baptism by fire." Dr. Conrad explained that one of her biggest fears about medical school was losing her sense of self because of the amount of work:

> Yeah; the workload is—it is pretty extreme. And I think because of [my] having had some other life experience[s], I also knew what it meant to maintain a balance, and not just only be a bookworm. And that piece, I think, is really important when we're looking at what is that workload, and how do you also end up maintaining a sense of self while you're in medical school?
>
> And I guess that's probably the biggest fear that I had: that I would lose my sense of self while I was there, because of all the workload. And for me, it was pretty much nonstop studying, and the hours were just incredibly intense. (Interview, December 8, 2019)

Most doctors enjoy medical school, despite (or perhaps because of) the hard work, and they connect the intense studies to the formation of social bonds with their peers. Dr. Susan Massey explained her medical school experience at University of Connecticut School of Medicine in 1990.

> Med school is—it's different than other education. There were one hundred of us (about), and we take the same classes every day, and we learn the same things every day. And then you study and interact with those people all the time. That was it. [Laughs.] It wasn't like I was going off to biology class, and someone is going off to their history class. It was—we all had the same class. And it really bonds you to this kind of whole group—you get to know each other pretty well.
>
> And it was a very routine thing. We had sort of desks in the anatomy lab. So, the first year we did gross anatomy (like typical medical school). And we could go back and just study in those labs; so, you had a subset of kids— maybe twelve of us would be in the same area (we might have desks near each other), and we would study.
>
> So, I would, you know, have classes all morning, all afternoon; go home and eat some cheese and crackers and then go back and hang out and study. (Interview, November 5, 2019)

Dr. Massey, however, also recalled feeling isolated from the wider society and important global events, such as the beginning of Desert Storm. "I remember the other thing that happened during that year of gross anatomy, in that lab (late at night) was when Desert Storm started. The war started, and we were all in there together, watching that. And kind of feeling a little spun out from the world in medical school" (interview, November 5, 2019).

Dr. Karen Ingram, who attended medical school at Duke University explained: "The first year was, kind of the classic phrase, probably everywhere (at least in medicine), was, it's like drinking from a firehose: there was so much all the time, all day long, with very little break from the book part.

"But it engenders a lot of comradery. . . . Probably my best friends now are from med school, from my previous timeframe, in my learning years" (Interview, February 13, 2020).

In addition to studying for classes, students must also study for and pass the United States Medical Licensing Exam (USMLE), which is administered in three parts (Step 1, Step 2, and Step 3) over a number of years. All MDs in the United States must pass all three Steps in order to apply for an unrestricted license to practice. Step 1 is taken after the second year of medical school. It is an eight-hour exam and covers knowledge of the basic sciences, which is why most medical students take their basic science classes within the first two years. The score students obtain on Step 1 is very important as a high Step 1 score is critical for placement into selective residency programs (residency is the next step in physician training after medical school). Medical students and residents spend a great deal of time and effort studying for Step exams since schools usually do not teach to the exam or offer specific training to pass it. According to July 2023 data from the National Board of Medical Examiners (NBME) website, it cost $660 to take the Step 1 exam in 2023.

The second two years of medical school are characterized by increasing clinical experience and exposure to patients on rotations, where students rotate through a variety of specialties for a specific period of time in order to learn about that specialty. Rotations expose students to nearly all aspects of medicine. Students usually have some choice as to which rotations they complete, and each rotation is organized according to its own internal logic. For example, a student might do a psychiatry rotation for a period of three weeks, while a surgical rotation might take several months. Rotations usually take place in hospitals, which may be private or public, such as a Veterans Administration hospital.

Rotations also are where hands-on, experiential-style learning that characterizes the heart of medical training exists. Dr. Ian Warner, a general surgeon, explained that he began learning to tie knots in medical school:

As a medical student, I would practice tying surgical knots with dental floss. I had a big box of floss (one of the big canisters), and I'd just pull off a yard (or so) at a time, and tie it around something and just start throwing knots. And so, you just learn how to—I practiced with my hands.

In fact, one of my surgical attendings, as a student, wanted me to try and tie a different knot, because there are different ways to tie knots, and you can use two hands or one hand. And I'd learned the one-handed technique.

And he's like, "I want you to do the two-handed technique." [Laughs.] And I'm like, "Uhh." So, I tried. And I hadn't practiced that, so I fumbled quite a bit. I'm like, "I don't understand why you want me to do this, but whatever."

But it was good, you know, it's good to know all of it. (Interview, January 13, 2020)

Students also learn to take responsibility for their patients during the third and fourth years, although they are supervised closely by other residents, fellows, attendings, and medical staff. They take histories, research their patients' conditions, and suggest diagnoses and courses of treatment. They report their findings and ideas to their superiors in staff conferences called "rounds," where they also receive feedback and critique. Medical schools also often have a research component to them, so in addition to doing rotations during their third and fourth years, students may conduct medical research or experiments.

During this time, students decide what branch of medicine they will pursue, and well-developed stereotypes about particular specialties circulate among medical students (see chap. 5). Some students enter their clinical years expecting to enjoy a particular specialty, only to discover that they actually want to do something else. Dr. Conrad, for example, was originally interested in psychiatry but did not enjoy her psychiatry rotations and so decided to go into pediatrics. At the last minute, however, she attended a psychiatry lecture at the advice of a mentor, and as she explained, "When I saw the neuroimages that this lector was discussing, I knew that that's where I needed to be. . . . And I changed all my applications that night, and started to pursue psychiatry again" (interview, December 8, 2019).

Students take Step 2 of the USMLE exam during their fourth year of medical school. Step 2 historically was a two-part exam. The first part is a nine-hour exam that cost approximately $660 in 2023 (according to the NBME website in July 2023) and tests students' knowledge of the clinical sciences (i.e., knowledge of various medical specialties that presumably they have learned on their rotations). The second part, which was suspended in 2020 due to COVID-19 and has since been eliminated, tested students' clinical skills by having them examine and diagnose a "patient" (in reality, an actor posing as a patient). The Step 2 clinical skills portion was only administered at five locations across the country. It cost $1,300 to take it in 2020, and students traveled to a given location in order to take the exam.

The Match

If the white coat ceremony is an opening ritual for medical school, then "the match"—the residency selection process—is the closing one. Students spend the final (fourth) year of medical school not only doing rotations but also applying for residency programs, which is the next step in their training. Residencies provide in-depth training within a particular specialty. Physicians must complete the first year of residency training (called the internship year) at minimum in order to obtain a license, but most doctors complete full residencies and may even complete more training beyond residency in the form of a fellowship or multiple subfellowships.

Like getting into medical school, obtaining a residency spot is a stressful and competitive process. Most medical students get one, but residency spots are not guaranteed since there are not enough spots to accommodate all medical students, and so fear of failure continues to haunt students as they seek residency. In 2019, for example, there were 43,000 applicants for 31,000 positions, but improvements have been made since that time. In 2023, there were 42,952 applicants of which 34,822 matched.[6] The shortage of residency spots means that at the end of medical school, students have no idea what type of doctor they will become until they actually obtain a residency spot in that specialty. Furthermore, many residencies are highly competitive. Some students do not get the type of residency they want and so are forced to go into another field.

Students first decide what specialties they want to pursue and then research which residency programs match their interests. Residency programs exist across the United States, and although they often are associated with large teaching hospitals, they also include rural areas and community hospitals. Students normally apply to their chosen residency programs through an application process organized by the National Resident Matching Program (NRMP).[7] Most students apply to programs across the country, and they usually apply to more than one type of residency in order to increase their chances of getting a spot. A student may apply to a number of dermatology residency programs as their first choice of specialty, for example, but as dermatology is highly competitive they may also apply for spots in less competitive programs, such as internal medicine, psychiatry, and family medicine in order to increase their chances of being placed.

Once the applications are completed in September of the fourth year, students receive an invitation by the residency program for an in-person interview if they are deemed competitive.[8] Interviews are scheduled between October and January, although each program interviews according to its own timeline. M4s travel at their own expense all over the country for interviews and some students interview at as many as six to ten places if they feel it is necessary.

Both applicants and residency programs then rank their preferences for admission. The medical student ranks residency programs in their order of preference, while residency programs rank their order of preference of interviewees in what are called "rank order lists." These ranked lists are submitted to the NRMP to make what is called a "match," that is, a match between an applicant and a program. The NRMP matches applicants with programs using a complicated mathematical algorithm based on research that was awarded a 2012 Nobel Prize in the Economic Sciences. The simplest match scenario is one in which a residency program in Texas lists applicant John Smith as its first preference, while John Smith also lists that program in Texas as his first choice, although reality is much more complicated (National Resident Matching Program, accessed July 5, 2023).

There is significant lag time between when the rank orders are submitted to the NRMP in January and when students find out whether or not they have "matched" in March. This three-month period is a time of heightened anxiety for students, anxiety that continues to increase until the third week of March, known as "Match Week." On Monday of Match Week, students learn whether or not they have matched but not where specifically. Students who did not match immediately begin a second matching process, known as the Supplemental Offer and Acceptance Program (SOAP, but colloquially known as the "scramble"), whereby they "scramble" to obtain a match in any residency program anywhere in the country that may, for whatever reason, still have an open spot. This process can be chaotic and may be considered humiliating, since a program with unfilled residency spots conveys the (not necessarily accurate) message that the program is of poor quality. Moreover, students who scramble are unlikely to obtain a spot in their specialty of choice. They are forced to give up their dream of becoming a certain kind of physician and to accept the reality that they are on a different, presumably lower-level career path. Students unable even to obtain a spot through SOAP are crushed and face difficult decisions about their immediate future.

The most important day of Match Week is Friday, also known as Match Day or "black Friday." This is the day that medical students across the nation find out with which residency program they have matched. The event is highly stressful in large part because the match is binding. Students must accept their residency match and begin training wherever they end up: they have no choice in the matter. The match completely determines the students' futures, including not only what type of doctor they will become, but also where they will live, the quality of their training, and what their working life will be like for the next three to seven years, a situation completely unique to medicine and unimaginable in any other profession.[9]

The way in which M4s find out where they "matched" varies from school to school. Many schools have a Match Day ceremony, providing ritual closure to the medical school experience. In 2004, Indiana University Medical School held a formal banquet. After the dinner, each student was called up by name and handed an envelope containing their match information. The student opened the envelope and announced to their fellow students where they had matched. Students who matched with their top or preferred residency programs were joyous and relieved, while students who matched with their less preferred programs or who suddenly discovered they were going into their second or third choice of medical fields were quieter and more reserved. Today, students receive their match notifications via email before any ceremony and so the surprise is not as public as it once was. All students who have matched begin preparing for their new lives as interns and residents, which starts annually across the country on July 1.

Internship and Residency

Once a student has matched, they begin residency training. Many residencies last three or four years. Ophthalmology, obstetrics-gynecology, neurology, dermatology, anesthesiology, and psychiatry, for example, are all four years, while internal medicine, family medicine, pediatrics, and emergency medicine last three years. Surgical residencies last at least five years. Further, many specialties have subspecialties that require additional fellowship training: if one wants to go into geriatrics, for example, one must first complete a family medicine or internal medicine residency, followed by a one or two year fellowship in geriatrics.

Residencies developed in the late nineteenth century out of a need for doctors to have more practical, experiential training beyond medical school. The first formal residency program was founded at John Hopkins, which established the nation's first scientific medical school in 1893. John Hopkins Hospital opened in 1889 and, following the German model of medical education, situated advanced clinical training within a university setting and applied university-based principles of research to hospital settings. The hospital at John Hopkins was considered to be a kind of graduate school and indeed, the main goal of the early Hopkins residency training was to prepare physicians for further education and research, with clinical training being a secondary goal (Ludmerer 2014, 22). When the hospital opened in 1889, it had a resident in medicine, surgery, and gynecology, and it soon added residents to additional fields (17). Residents at Hopkins lived in the hospital for years as they completed what was understood as a kind of institutional apprenticeship (20). The term *residency* therefore is derived from this time period when physicians were male, usually unmarried, and expected to actually live at the hospital (also called the "house") in which they worked—that is, they were a "resident" of the house. Trainees were expected to devote themselves day and night to their work, an expectation that continues in modified form today. This attitude toward work is summarized in the statements made by Dr. William Osler, one of the founders of the John Hopkins residency program who, when asked about a physician's duties toward his family, responded: "Leave them! Heavy as are your responsibilities to those nearest and dearest, they are outweighed by the responsibilities to yourself, to the profession, and to the public" (quoted in Ludmerer 2014, 91).

This model of residency and Osler's perspective on resident work hours eventually spread throughout the country. The early twentieth century witnessed the development of "internships," where post–medical school graduates gained additional clinical experience through an additional year of training; by the 1930s, most medical school graduates completed internships and many state licensure boards deemed them important for training (Howell 2016). After World War II, residencies became even more common as physicians sought to specialize and hospitals came to rely on resident labor.

Most new residents move to another city or state to begin residency. Residents are paid employees, although their salary is considered low for physicians: the average incoming salary for a first-year resident in 2022 was $58,700, but that figure varies widely by residency program, specialty, and location. Specialties such as internal medicine, family medicine, and emergency medicine tend to draw lower salaries, while specialties such as surgery, critical care, and immunology are higher. Such salaries seem high but should be considered alongside the amount of student debt residents carry, which they begin to repay at this time. In 2022, medical school debt was above $300,000 for 26 percent of residents, while another 24 percent carried somewhere between $200,000 and $300,000 in student loans for the same year. Another 22 percent, however, carried no debt at all (Robbins 2022).

Terminology regarding residencies can be confusing. The term *resident* is short for "resident physician"; however, the first year of residency is called an "internship," and first-year residents often are known as "interns" or colloquially as "'terns." Residents also may be called "house officers," "officers," or "senior house officers"—the last if they are in their final year of residency. The term *officer* likely originated from health officers serving in the military. They also may be called junior or senior residents depending on their year, or the terms PG1 (postgraduate year 1), PG2, and PG3 may be used to refer to first-, second-, and third-year residents. Collectively, residents may be referred to as "housestaff," "house" being a colloquial term for hospital. Finally, the term *chief* usually refers to a resident who has extended their residency for an additional year in order to gain more administrative and supervisory experience within a specialty.

The intern year, or first year of residency, is one of the most strenuous years in terms of work and tends to be a year in which a lot of folklore emerges. Interns have little status or authority, and they are responsible for doing the majority of low-level work (sometimes called "scut work"), which in the past consisted of minor tasks like drawing blood and today consists of filling out forms and doing administrative paperwork (Howell 2016, 130). Interns do not set their own schedules, and they often work holidays and weekends for the entire year, often with very little sleep and few days (or nights) off. The well-known book *The House of God*, published in 1978 by Samuel Shem is a fictionalized satire of Shem's own intern year (1973–74) at Beth Israel Hospital in Boston. The book unflinchingly portrays the terrible working conditions, lack of sleep, and psychological trauma interns endured at that time (including the suicide of one intern). The depictions of intern life were so controversial that the book originally was banned by medical school deans. Although a work of fiction, Shem/Bergman has stated in print that it is a largely authentic account of his experience (Bergman 2019, 486) and writes that, at the time, "gallows humor was the currency of our relationship" largely to deal with "our impotence in the face of human suffering" (NYU Langone Health 2019 at 15:20).

Working conditions for residents have improved since Shem's time, but the intern year remains quite difficult. Shem's book continues to be popular among medical students and residents and has sold over three million copies. The user comments that accompanied Shem/Bergman's reflections on *The House of God* on the fortieth anniversary of its publication illustrate that the experiences described in the book continue to resonate.

July 13, 2019
.Loved the Book
Gordon Banks, MD |
I first read the book as a student in 1977. We were told it would make us
cynical, but if you trained at an inner-city hospital, you already were. I'd say
the book helped us keep our sanity under stressful conditions of internship.

July 15, 2019
People Remain The Same, Technology Moves On
Robert Mulcahy, MD | Retired, Lake Health System
The patients, caregivers, financial interests, personalities, strains, conflicts,
victories and defeats are all as identifiable in today's medical environment as
they were in *The House of God.*

July 11, 2019
So Timely
Marni Friedman, MD | Private Practice
I just so happen to be halfway through a re-reading of this classic, having
picked it up again after 20 or more years. The details of life on the wards
bring my training years back to me vividly—the emotions, the smells, the
battle for sleep and sanity—despite the fact my residency was a decade and
a half after the depicted era. (Bergman 2019)

Today, there are a plethora of how-to guides geared toward helping incoming
interns navigate the year. With titles like "Tips from the Trenches" and "Medical Intern Survival Guide," these publications make it clear that the intern year
remains something to be survived.

It is difficult to describe a typical day of residency since each day varies
and residency experiences differ according to specialty and program. A day
often begins with morning rounds, which may start anywhere between 4:00
a.m. and 7:00 a.m. The term *rounds* refers to the daily visits to patients by that
patient's main physician and the care team. Rounds are a form of experiential
learning for everyone involved. They are designed to teach interns and residents
about conditions and diseases; they also are a structured forum for deciding
the best plan of care for the patient. Rounds may be done at the patient's bed
in a hospital, or they may be done without the patient present in a conference
room. Often it is the job of the intern, who presumably has the least amount of
medical knowledge, to check on the patient first, see how they are doing, learn
about the patient's condition, and conduct research about what the next steps
might be. Most interns and residents arrive at the hospital well before rounds
in order to prepare. Interns learn to present their patients as "cases," meaning

that information such as changes in the patient's condition or any additional information that the intern has found is presented in a highly formalized and systematic way (Anspach 1988).[10] Dr. Warner described rounds during his surgical residency:

> The hours could be crazy. The rotations—some of the rotations were more intensive, and so I'd get up at three o'clock in the morning and start my rounds before the attendings would come in at six thirty, or six, or five forty-five, or whenever they decided to come in, before we started surgery at seven-thirty.
>
> So, I had to have all the patients seen and rounded on, and labs checked, and make sure that things were where they should be. And the attendings would come in, and I would have to present everybody, and then we'd go through and round with them.
>
> So, there [were] a few months where I felt like it was more arduous, because I was working from three until (sometimes) seven or eight at night, and get home (maybe) eight or nine, say hi to my family real quick, try and get some sleep, [laughing] go back and do it again. (Interview, January 13, 2020)

Rounds are led by a senior resident, fellow, or attending physician, and the intern is asked questions or may be challenged on their information and presumptions. Interns and residents also attend "grand rounds," which are more formal lectures and conferences that take place throughout the year and are usually open to the entire medical community of the hospital. Grand rounds might consist of a formal presentation or lecture by an invited speaker, a presentation of new research and technology, or a discussion/debate of a current ethical issue.

Residents also start learning their specialty in much greater detail and with much more precision during this time. Dr. Warner described:

> **IW:** You start by doing the tasks that you can't mess up. [Laughs.] So, watching is the first one. So, as a student you do a lot of watching, and then you retract, which actually is probably harder than some of the other things that they would have us do. You know, as you move up you realize that it's really easy to mess up retracting and not know.
>
> And then you learn how to close the skin, so you put sutures in, and you try to close the skin up, and dress the incision. So, as you get more proficient, then you get the next task, and the next task.
>
> But for us, in our [residency] program, there [were] enough people ahead of you that you really didn't do much operating until your third

year, probably. And then you started doing some of the smaller cases, you know?

As a second-year resident, you probably would do some of the really small cases.

LG: What would be an example of a small case?

IW: Maybe if you had a lipoma, which is a little fatty mass; it usually sits in the subcutaneous tissue, so right under the skin there is a layer of fat. And these tend to grow in that area. It's really hard to mess those up, and so you start by doing stuff like that.

And so, you get to make the incision, you get to pull the tumor out, and then you get to close the incision. And so, you get to the whole thing yourself—which is great when you're first, "Oh, I get to do something."

But as you get further along, you want bigger things, you want to do more. And so, that continues as you move through the years, you get bigger and bigger cases, until you know, your fourth and fifth year you're doing a majority of the surgery; often, in conjunction with your attending physician. . . . But [the attending] is also guiding me. It's like, "Don't cut that; oh, stop, back up." You know, and just kind of correcting me as I tried to sabotage through surgery. . . . One of our attendings would call us "the first combatants" instead of the first assistants. (Interview, January 13, 2020)

The long work long hours and lack of sleep that characterize residency are formalized through "call schedules." The term *call* or *being on call* means that a physician is available to work after his or her regular work has ended. Residents on call take care of all patients, not just their own, so they are responsible for more patients than during their normal workday. They also are responsible for any new patient admissions (sometimes called "hits") that come in during their call. Call, therefore, is often quite busy, characterized by little sleep or time to eat. Residents may get no sleep on call, or on "good nights"—meaning the hospital is slow—they may sleep several hours if there is not much work to do. On call, residents' sleep is inversely proportionate to the care required by patients.

Many residencies have a call schedule of one in three (q3) or one in four (q4) nights (the abbreviation q means "every"). Some surgical residencies have call every other night (q2). Most on-call residents are required to be physically in the hospital. The following is an example of a q3 call schedule taken from an internal medicine residency when the resident was working in the ICU (intensive care unit):

- Day 1 of call: Begin regular workday at approximately 6:30 a.m. Two teams take admissions from 7:00 a.m. on, and the "short call" team signs out around 5:00 p.m. The overnight team stays in the hospital, working throughout the night. The intern/resident may get some sleep if it is a slow night, but often sleeps as little as half an hour or not at all if it is a busy night.

- Day 2 of call: Finish call in the morning and transition patients to the on-call team after rounds (or on rounds if rounds run longer than sign-out time).

- Day 3 of call: Begin regular workday around 6:30 a.m. Work full day and go home sometime in the evening.

- Repeat call schedule beginning with Day 1.

Pediatric surgeon Dr. Doug Corgain described his q2 schedule during his surgery residency at the University of Michigan in the mid-1990s.

> So, I did five years of clinical surgery as a general surgery resident, plus two years of research, and then two years of pediatric surgery residency. And back then, much of that was on call every other night. . . . That means there is always a resident surgeon in-house. And the way we staffed the services then, there were two of us at any level. So, in your early years, it means every other day you sleep in the hospital. And the days you're not sleeping in the hospital, you work all day. So: come in Monday morning, work all day Monday, stay Monday night, work all day Tuesday, go home about six or seven o'clock at night on Tuesday. Sleep in your own bed Tuesday night. Get up, come in Wednesday, do the same thing until Thursday evening. So, it is super intense. (Interview, December 19, 2019)

Dr. Brian Price, an orthopedic surgeon, described his residency experience:

> Orthopedic residency was really hard. It's a lot of kind of really long hours, a lot of kind of physical and mental challenges.
> I remember the first weekend of call I took, they call them "super Saturdays," where you're like an intern, covering the pager for kind of the Children's Hospital and Barnes Hospital, which is—I mean, it's—the hospital is huge, it's, I don't know, a mile or two across.
> So, you would be handed the pager at seven o'clock in the morning, and then you'd be covering all the consult calls, all the floor calls, as well as some of the patient calls in (for their attendings). . . . So, I mean your pager would just be going off all day. . . .

So, you'd be seeing consults in the ER [emergency room]; seeing floor consults, dealing with floor patients, dealing with phone calls from, you know, patients that had had surgery, from pharmacies—it was just like—it was really like drinking from a firehose. And it would be like thirty hours of nonstop—. . . Just nonstop action.

I remember at the end of your super Saturday, you'd just be soaked in sweat and exhausted. [Chuckling.] And then but you know, I think it was good to be able to learn how to manage and prioritize, you know, different things. So, you know, you'd just have to learn what was urgent and what you could put on a back burner, and what, you know, what had to be addressed right away. (Interview, November 8, 2019)

Some residencies, such as that for internal medicine, may also require "night float," which is where residents work nights rather than days for a set period of time, perhaps one week every month. The purpose of night float is to free up other residents so that they can sleep on a more regular schedule and do less call by having more doctors regularly available at night.

Call schedules, night float, and the never-ending nature of work can make maintaining personal relationships difficult for residents. Several physicians I talked to found residency isolating from people who were not associated with the hospital, such as their family and wider society as a whole. Work and patient relationships, however, may be intense. Dr. Corgain observed,

I think it's a time where, by virtue of being in the hospital that much, you've got really a particular and special relationship with your patients. Even though they realize you're the junior doctor, and that you're not making the final decisions, they—in a big university hospital like that—the patients realize you're the one that's there all the time, and kind of come to trust you as the factfinder and the person that can navigate the system for them. So, I think you know, then with the nurses—you're there all the time, so you're their go-to person. And then if you're receptive, and listen, and learn from them, they become friends. So, it was really exhausting, really tiring time; but also, pretty special. (Interview, December 19, 2019)

It was not until 2003 that the ACGME, under pressure from the Occupational and Safety Health Administration, introduced the controversial concept of "resident duty hours," which limited the number of hours residents were allowed to work. Prior to 2003, there were no restrictions on resident duty hours: residents worked all the time, well over one hundred hours a week, a practice based on the John Hopkins model. Under the 2003 regulations, residents were supposed to work no more than eighty hours per week averaged over four weeks; were required to have one day off in seven; and were to have at least eight hours off between shifts (see DeZee et al. 2012:524; Doolittle 2017). Second- and third-year residents could work no more than twenty-four hours in a row with an additional four hours allotted for transition time and education. Interns originally were limited to sixteen hours in a row, although in 2017 interns were put on the same duty hour limitations as other residents.

The implementation of resident duty hours restrictions was controversial and remains so today. One of the arguments for having unlimited work hours is that residency is the primary period during which physicians learn, and one must learn all one can during this time. Indeed, one common medical saying is "The only thing wrong with being on call every other night is that you only get to see half the cases." This saying refers to the idea that those doctors who are not on call are missing out on valuable experiences, and it illustrates how internship and residency socialize physicians into a perspective in which work is prioritized above everything else. Another argument against limiting workplace hours is the fact that when one enters private practice, there is no such thing as limited work hours: patients require attention day or night, and so a rigorous work schedule accustoms doctors to working at all hours. As Dr. Warner observed regarding his post-residency work experience, "It [the workload] hasn't changed a lot. I don't have anybody to do my work for me now, so it's all me" (interview, January 13, 2020). A third argument is that such a work schedule is consistent with good patient care because patients have the same physician for longer periods of time, and physicians learn more about the particular details of the patients themselves. Shorter periods of work entail multiple transitions between care providers, leading to an increase in errors.

Advocates of resident duty hour restrictions point out that sleep-deprived residents make more mistakes and put patient safety at risk; physician well-being is cited as a secondary, more minor concern. One commonly cited sleep deprivation study used to support resident duty hours was conducted on employees in the transportation industry and in the army. It showed few differences between a person who had not slept in twenty-eight hours and a person who was intoxicated with a blood level of .10 (Williamson and Feyer 2000). Other studies, however, show that resident duty hour regulations had little impact on patient care outcomes or on resident well-being. Some even indicated that limited duty hours might negatively affect residents and increase burnout, since residents had less time to attend teaching conferences and the intensity of their workload increased with the reduction in hours—that is, the amount of work remained the same, while only the hours had been reduced (Doolittle 2017). Further, some of my interviewees who completed residency after work duty hour restrictions were implemented said that they simply fibbed about the number of hours they worked in order to comply with the requirement. The reality is that despite formal regulation, residents continue to work long hours.

Step 3 of the USMLE typically is taken after intern year. Step 3 is a two-day exam that assesses a resident's ability to apply medical knowledge and the clinical sciences in order to enter unsupervised medical practice. The first day of the exam is approximately seven hours and the second day is approximately nine hours. Once a person passes Step 3, he or she may apply for a medical license from the state licensing agency. In some states, MDs may apply for a medical license after passing Step 3 and completed the intern year; other states, however, require completion of a full residency in order to obtain a medical license. Once residency is completed and a physician has obtained a medical license from the state licensing board, they may formally begin unsupervised medical practice. Physicians are required to provide evidence of continuing education to retain their license, usually about fifty hours per year (DeZee et al. 2012).

Fellowship and Beyond

Physicians wanting more specialization within a medical field complete a fellowship after residency. The main purpose of a fellowship is to obtain additional training and knowledge, and many subspecialties require fellowships. Like residencies, the length of fellowships depends on the field, but they can last between one and five years. Orthopedic surgery, for example, entails a five-year residency, and then to become a hand surgeon, one must complete an additional year of a hand fellowship. To become a heart surgeon, one must first complete a residency in general surgery, which lasts five years, and then do a two- or three-year fellowship in cardiovascular surgery. A cardiologist, on the other hand, must complete a three-year residency in internal medicine and then three years of a cardiology fellowship, plus, if necessary, a subspecialty fellowship (such as echocardiography) that may last one or two years. Fellows have more status and authority than residents and supervise them in addition to their regular work. The life of a fellow is not easy, however, and consists of much of the same schedule as residencies, including call schedules and working weekends and holidays. Fellows may also do medical research as part of their fellowship.

Many physicians choose to take board exams in order to become "board certified" in their specialties. A board-certified physician means that the doctor is practicing at the very highest level of expertise in their specialty; it is an exam that "certifies" that the doctor's knowledge and skills are up to date. Some board certifications are taken right after residency, like internal medicine boards. Subspecialty boards such as critical care or pulmonology are not taken until after fellowship is competed. Highly trained physicians might obtain several board certifications. A physician who has completed an internal medicine residency and completed a fellowship in pulmonary/critical care, for example, can become board certified in internal medicine, pulmonary disease, and critical care medicine, thus being triple board certified. Board certification is not required: a physician may successfully complete a residency in internal medicine but may choose not to take internal medicine boards. In the era of increasing specialization, however, many physicians choose to become board certified and many insurance carriers require their physicians to be board certified to be credentialed.[11]

Conclusion

The road to becoming a physician is characterized by years of study, hard work, financial debt, and sacrifice. It also is characterized by delay. Physicians tend to delay relationships, marriage, and children, perhaps buying a first house in their thirties and sometimes beyond. Orthopedic surgeon Dr. Price said, "Your friends are kind of starting their careers, and buying homes, and kind of starting their life. . . . where[as] your life is just kind of on hold. . . . That was probably the hardest thing" (interview, November 8, 2019). The result is that physicians completely and fully internalize hard work and their identity as a doctor. If the world of work and professional training might be compared to a footrace, physicians are the ultrarunners.

It is true that the medical work environment also has changed significantly in the past twenty years and that it continues to evolve. The implementation of resident duty hours, however controversial, has increased public awareness of the problematic number of hours worked. Medicine also is more patient centered than it was in the past, and many programs are more supportive of staff needs. The influx of women in the twenty-first century, the influence of evidence-based medicine, the use of electronic medical records (EMRs), and the increasing use of team-based approaches all continue to affect how physicians are trained and medical work is organized, and these are significant shifts from how medicine was practiced in the twentieth century.

But it also remains true that medical training continues to exact a toll on practitioners. Doctors are trained to work no matter what, including at the expense of their own physical comfort and limitations and sometimes at the cost of relationships and family. The training teaches physicians to be tough and self-reliant, but it also discourages them from asking for help or from admitting they are tired or sick. Workaholism is common (one might argue even culti-vated and rewarded), and the abuse of alcohol, drugs, and sex exists, although there few studies address such problems directly (see chap. 2). In sum, while there is no doubt that it is a great achievement to become a doctor, doing so comes at a cost. That cost is examined in more detail in the next chapter.

Notes

1. There are two types of medical schools. Allopathic medical schools are conventional medical schools that utilize a standard science-based curriculum, while osteopathic schools offer a more holistic approach, including complementary and alternative medical practices such as spinal manipulation and massage therapy.

2. The acceptance rate is the number of applications an institution accepts, while the admittance rate is the number of students who actually matriculate into the institution.

3. The demographic statistics I have included do not include mixed ethnic categories such as "Hispanic, Latino, or of Spanish Origin," "Black or African American," or other federally designated "mixed" categories.

4. Wikipedia, s.v., "Declaration of Geneva," last edited 16 November, 2023, https://en.wikipedia.org/wiki/Declaration_of_Geneva.

5. While nearly all medical schools have a white coat ceremony, whether physicians actually wear a white coat depends on the specific institutional cul-ture. Arguments against wearing the white coat state that all the white coat does is reinforce hierarchies and actually contributes to disease by carrying germs, while others argue that patients actually prefer the white coat as it symbolizes authority and is what patients expect. For details on these arguments, see Hochberg 2007.

6. The reason there is a shortage of residency spots is complex and has to do with the way medical school and graduate medical education is funded. Gradu-ate medical education (residency) is subsidized through Medicare. Increasing the number of residency spots would entail changes to the way in which Medi-care is organized and funded, a difficult and highly politicized topic.

7. Not all residency programs participate in the match, but most of them do. Each residency program has its own requirements and preferences, and appli-cants must meet basic eligibility criteria to be considered for a match.

8. The information outlined in this chapter pertains to the main match program and not the specialty program match or the match for international applicants, both of which are different programs.

9. The match is binding only for the first year of the residency program. Whether or not a physician continues in their residency depends on their performance as evaluated by the residency program.

10. Renee Anspach (1988) analyzed the language of case presentations, noting that typical case presentations use passive voice and depersonalize the patient by separating biological processes from the person and making technology seem like an active agent.

11. The cost to apply to take boards in 2023 was $750–$800, and the cost to actually take the exam varied by specialty. The internal medicine exam cost was $1,950, while the cost of the exam for anesthesiology was $1,400, plus an additional $1,600 for an oral exam in 2022. Physicians travel to designated locations at their own expense to take boards.

2

"Living the Dream"

Suffering, Moral Injury, and Trauma in Medical Practice

A common saying used by physicians in residency training is that they are "living the dream." Superficially this phrase refers to the power, wealth, status, and respect associated with the job: that is, to be a physician means living out the American dream of financial and social success. But the phrase is ironic, and physicians only tell each other they are "living the dream" when their working situation is burdensome, unpleasant, or even intolerable.

This chapter explores why doctoring is difficult and suggests that physicians suffer as a result of their work. It is commonly understood that the medical community seeks to reduce suffering in patients, but it is less commonly recognized that medical professionals can suffer as well. Physicians do not usually see themselves as people who suffer because their work is focused on their patients. Yet in interviews physicians admitted that they sometimes suffered because of work, and when I asked them what the most difficult or challenging thing was about being a doctor, they often responded with a story, some of which are shared here.

Physician suffering is important for several reasons. First, acknowledging it may lead to relief through practical measures because physician suffering is downplayed, overlooked, or recast as something else, such as burnout, or a problem of resilience, hindering opportunities to provide appropriate correctives. Second, physician suffering is important because suffering is a cultural feature of medicine, not merely a clinical one. As a cultural feature, suffering is constitutive of medical practice, extending beyond the practical problem of its alleviation. Patients suffer; caretakers suffer; and caretakers are tasked with the job of relieving suffering. Acknowledging suffering as constitutive advances understanding of medicine. Finally, physician suffering is important because it constitutes the deep context for the medical carnivalesque.

It is important to state that just because physicians may suffer does not mean that they do not enjoy being physicians. Most physicians love their work and find it gratifying. They worked hard to become a doctor, and it is a crucial aspect of their identity. Nor does it mean that they suffer extensively, as much as patients do, or all the time. But it is entirely possible both to love one's work and to endure a certain degree of suffering: these are not mutually exclusive. Further, to state that care providers suffer in no way diminishes the importance of patient suffering. Patient suffering is the reason medicine exists, and physicians are the first people to acknowledge that. However, as Katie Watson (2011, 38) writes, "Surely we can advocate for the humanity of patients without denying the humanity of those who treat them."

Physician Suicide

The most concrete evidence that physicians suffer is the extraordinarily high suicide rate. Physicians have one of the highest suicide rates of any occupation, with a death by suicide rate twice that of active military members (Symon 2018; Talbot and Dean 2018).[1] The most commonly cited statistic is that there are about four hundred physician suicides per year, which is the equivalent of approximately two incoming medical school classes.[2] One of my conversational partners, anesthesiologist Dr. Mark York at the University of Utah, characterized physician suicide as a national epidemic (interview, September 6, 2018). A second conversational partner mentioned he had at least four colleagues commit suicide. Physician-authors have written about suicide as well: Abraham Verghese's bestselling memoir *The Tennis Partner* (1998), for example, detailed one physician's struggle with addiction that ended in suicide.

Female physicians are particularly at risk. The suicide rate is 250–400 percent higher among female physicians as compared to women in other professions, while for male physicians the suicide rate is 70 percent higher when compared to other professional men (Brunk 2015; see also Caan 2019; Bailey, Robinson, and McGorry 2018). Among surgeons, suicide ideation is reported at a rate of about 1:16 (Shanafelt et al. 2011).

Physician suicide and risk of suicide are not limited to doctors in the United States. Global physician suicide has a standardized mortality ratio of 1.44 (Dutheil et al. 2019), making physician suicide an occupational issue rather than one associated with nationality or region. Finland, Norway, Australia, and China all have conducted studies on physician suicide rates, although rates are not uniform. The US has a higher suicide rate than Europe, for example, where rates have declined for the past decade due to changes in how medicine is practiced (Dutheil et al. 2019), although it remains a problem. One Norwegian study analyzed physician deaths between the years 1960 and 2000 as compared to other human service occupations and the general population and found that doctors were at the highest risk for suicide (Hem et al. 2005). The study also concluded that female doctors were at a higher risk than men, with nearly 5 percent of all female physician deaths between 1960 and 2000 due to suicide. A follow-up study concluded that physicians in Norway had an overall lower mortality rate than the general population except when it came to suicide (Aasland et al. 2011). Studies in Australia also concluded that medical practitioners are at high risk for suicide (Bailey, Robinson, and McGorry 2018). Further, the problem of physician suicide appears long-lived: according to researchers Claudia Center and colleagues (2003), physicians in England observed a higher suicide rate among doctors as early as 1858. In the UK, it remains a problem: the annual UK local medical committees conference in Belfast passed a motion on March 19, 2019, in recognition of "the appalling statistics and circumstances of doctor suicides" (Iacobucci 2019).

Recognition of the problem of physician suicide is growing, but slowly. Researchers Daniel DeSole, Philip Singer, and Samuel Aronson (1969) published an early article that provided information on the number of suicides per year, but apperception began in earnest in the first decade of the twenty-first century with a working group organized by the American Foundation for Suicide Prevention (Center et al. 2003), which reviewed the extant literature on physician suicide and provided a consensus statement on research priorities and recommendations for reform. Almost two decades later, one scoping review presented as a poster at the American College of Physicians (ACP) Internal Medicine Meeting in 2019 reviewed 347 articles on physician suicide and concluded that there was still a lack of reliable, consistent information and that more research was needed (Campbell 2019). There also are at least two documentary films that deal with physician suicide specifically. *Struggling in Silence: Physician Depression and Suicide* was produced in 2008 by the American Foundation for Suicide Prevention and focused on destigmatizing mental health issues like depression among doctors. *Do No Harm*, released in 2017, focused on systemic problems in the health care system, including the massive competitiveness of medical school, crushing student debt, long work hours, sleep deprivation (particularly for interns and residents), unreasonable expectations, and the punitive nature of the system with respect to physician mental health. The film placed the blame squarely on the organization of medical work, characterizing the working conditions of doctors in teaching hospitals as abusive and potentially violating the United Nations Declaration of Human Rights (Symon 2018). One point both documentaries make is that physician suicide is not talked about: the word *silence* in the title of the documentary *Struggling in Silence* illustrates its taboo nature. As one interviewee states in *Do No Harm*, "It's [physician suicide] the dirty little secret that no one wants to talk about." Dr. Pamela Wible, an outspoken physician advocate and activist in the film, characterizes this lack of attention as a deliberate silencing or covering up of the issue.

Burnout, Moral Injury, Trauma, and Suffering

Physician distress, including suicide, most commonly is addressed through the framework of "burnout." I argue elsewhere that burnout is a euphemism for suffering (Gabbert 2020). Burnout is defined variously but includes criteria such as "overwhelming exhaustion, feelings of cynicism and detachment from the job, and a sense of ineffectiveness and lack of accomplishment" (Maslach and Leither 2016, 103). It also is characterized as "emotional exhaustion, depersonalization, and feelings of low achievement and decreased effectiveness" (Noseworthy et al. 2017). Burnout is not classified in the *DSM5* (fifth edition of the *Diagnostic and Statistical Manual of Mental Disorders*) as a psychiatric disorder, but it is indexed in the *ICD*-11 (eleventh revision of the International Statistical Classification of Diseases and Related Health Problems by the World Health Organization) as an occupational phenomenon resulting from chronic workplace stress.

Research on physician burnout has focused on developing measurements (such as the Maslach Burnout Inventory, the standard measurement), forming conceptual models, and building strategies for recovery and prevention, with a particular emphasis on increasing resilience (e.g., Epstein and Krasner 2013; Outram and Kelly 2014). The first statistical measurement of physician burnout in the US was conducted in 2012, which concluded that 45.8 percent of physicians reported at least one symptom (Shanafelt et al. 2012); a 2021 national report on physician burnout, depression, and suicide reported a slightly lower rate of 42 percent. Rates of burnout for female physicians were reported at 51 percent and for men 36 percent (Kane 2021).

Burnout has been called a "public health crisis" that "should be considered an early warning sign of dysfunction in our health care system" (Noseworthy et al. 2017). In 2015, it appeared to be getting worse rather than better (Shanafelt et al. 2015). According to one report, the increase in burnout was attributable to "loss of control over work, increased performance measurement (quality, cost, patient experience), the increasing complexity of medical care, the implementation of electronic health records (EHRs), and profound inefficiencies in the practice environment, all of which have altered work flows and patient interactions" (Noseworthy et al. 2017). Burnout is correlated with patient safety issues and medical error, which is the third-leading cause of death in the United States (Dutheil et al. 2019, 19). Burnout also is associated with cost issues, as it affects decisions about early retirement and part-time work and contributes to high turnover and reduced clinical effort (Noseworthy et al. 2017). Finally, burnout is associated with depression and suicide. Among surgeons, for example, burnout is correlated with physician impairment, including drug and alcohol abuse, suicidal ideation, and depression (Oreskovich et al. 2012).

The problem with the term *burnout*, however, is that it does not really address the sense of existential crisis that may accompany doctoring. A closer term is *moral injury*.[3] The concept of moral injury was coined by Dr. Jonathan Shay to characterize the psychological trauma and experiences of soldiers from the Vietnam War. The main webpage of the Shay Moral Injury Center as of July 6, 2023, described moral injury as "the suffering people experience when we are in high stakes situations, things go wrong, and harm results that challenges our deepest moral codes and ability to trust in others or ourselves. The harm may be something we did, something we witnessed, or something that was done to us. It results in moral emotions such as shame, guilt, self-condemnation, outrage, and sorrow." Moral injury is a form of trauma. The Greek root of the word *trauma* means a physical wound, but today the word also entails psychological ones.[4] Simon Talbot and Wendy Dean successfully applied the concept of moral injury to physicians, arguing in a 2018 op-ed that moral injury for doctors consisted of "being unable to provide high-quality care and healing in the context of health care" (2). They argued that physicians were not burning out, they were sustaining moral injuries that were a direct result of flaws in the health care system. Elements that contribute to moral injury over time are similar to those identified for burnout and include the role of insurance companies, increasing bureaucracy, excessive testing, EHRs, and the prioritization of speed and efficiency over time spent with patients (Bailey 2020). Cynda Rushton, a nurse and professor of clinical ethics at John Hopkins University who studied the related notion of "moral distress," states, "What both of these terms signify is *a sense of suffering* that clinicians are experiencing in their roles now, in ways that they haven't in the past" (Bailey 2020, italics mine).

Both burnout and moral injury describe provider suffering. Burnout is a manifestation of suffering, while moral injury is trauma that can lead to suffering. Suffering itself is difficult to quantify because it is a holistic, existential phenomenon that is difficult to define. The first general definition in the Oxford English Dictionary (OED) defined the verb form of suffering as "to undergo, endure," and immediately after, the first entry listed the transitive form as "to have (something painful, distressing, or injurious) inflicted or imposed upon one; to submit to with pain, distress, or grief."[5] Doctors deal with suffering in their ordinary work, but physicians historically equated pain with suffering due to the disease model that dominated medicine (further discussed in this chapter). They treated suffering by relieving pain. Even today the relief of pain dominates medical practice, with pain management clinics, analgesic medicines, and pain management plans that in some views contributed to the opioid epidemic.

Dr. Eric Cassell, a physician and ethicist, was one of the first clinicians to approach suffering from a holistic perspective in his influential 1991 book *The Nature of Suffering and the Goals of Medicine*. Cassell observed that patients could be in great physical pain but not necessarily suffer, leading him to theorize that suffering was a broader, more holistic phenomenon that entailed the mind, body, and spirit or, in his framework, "a person." Cassell called on physicians to treat suffering by treating the entire person and not just as a manifestation of a more general disease.

The reason Cassell argued for this approach is that, beginning in approximately the 1920s, physicians were trained according to a disease model of illness, a model that originated in nineteenth-century France. The disease model meant that different diseases were thought to have different origins and causes and that diseases manifested the same way in different individuals. The doctor's professional duty as a scientist was to find, explain, and then treat the disease (Faber in Cassell [1991] 2004, 6). This disease-based model privileged scientific and technical knowledge, replacing an earlier model that relied on the experience, personal knowledge, and skills of the physician to understand and treat illness. In the new scientific model, disease was abstracted from patients and it was diseases that were treated rather than sick persons. In advocating for a holistic model of healing, Cassell identified important components of suffering, including shame, isolation, a sense of powerlessness, a lack of hope, meaninglessness, and a perceived threat to personhood or identity. He also added, "No one has ever questioned the suffering that attends the loss of hope" (41).

Cassell targeted patient suffering, but his ideas are applicable to the experiences of care providers in the context of work. Threats to one's identity as a physician and work-related trauma such as moral injury accrue over time, and these may be compounded by social isolation, shame, or perceived powerlessness. Feelings of ineffectiveness or even meaninglessness, for example, begin for some people in medical school. Medical students are bright, motivated, somewhat idealistic young people who are accustomed to success. In medical school, they learn that many forms of health care delivery aren't necessarily what is best for the patient or even what the patient might want. The story that follows (which has been edited for readability), for example, was told to me by a second-year medical student about their rounds at a Veterans Administration (VA) hospital:

> So, there's a lot of patients at the VA. And it's really sad because our entire system is devised around test[s] and treatments; and yet, at the VA I'd say the majority of the chief complaints are centered [on] psychiatric concerns, especially in internal medicine—for males with service experience over the age of sixty-five. And what's really hard is, I've been doing like histories and people literally just start bawling; they're like, "Please, like I need to see somebody. Like, I want to, you know, end my life." They'll flat-out say that.
>
> And you'll report to your attending [physician], "The patient, you know, is suicidal and his ejection fraction is, you know, thirty-five." And they're like, "Oh, we've got to get this guy upstairs quick, you know, his ejection fraction is thirty-five. . . ."
>
> It's like the person has a problem that we can fix, and the person has, frankly, a problem that we can't fix, which is a psychiatric illness. . . .
>
> And the sad thing is, is so they'll put $100,000 of hardware in this guy, and he's going to come back three years later—he's going to be able to walk in from the parking lot, so it's a win for the surgeon upstairs. And he [the patient] goes, "All right, well I still can't forgive myself for the thirteen-year-old girl I shot when I was in Vietnam, and I still want to end my life." So, then you have to ask yourself, . . . What have we really done? (Anonymous, interview, March 21, 2012)

In this story, the vet was able to walk again because of a successful operation, but the health care system was unable to relieve his interior psychological pain, leaving him with suicidal thoughts. The student stated later that this was one of many examples they experienced, causing the student to question: "You have to ask yourself—What have we really done?" This questioning, along with the student's underlying sense of responsibility to help alleviate the vet's condition, caused distress and cognitive dissonance, threats to their identity and core beliefs.

Emergency room physician Dr. Maija Elonen recalled feelings of help-lessness and abandonment in medical school during a particularly difficult case:

In medical school I remember having this period with this same cystic fibrosis patient that I was taking care of. I was so involved with this guy that got flown from Alaska to get new lungs at UNC [University of North Carolina–Chapel Hill] (it's a big pulmonary service), and they saw a lot of cystic fibrosis.

He had gotten this lung transplant, and someone forgot to put an NG tube [nasogastric tube] down him, and he aspirated everything from his stomach— all the acid from his stomach—into his new transplanted lungs. But as a medical student, I can tell you like, this was horrible, it was a mistake: someone forgot to do this. But it took me a long time to figure out what was happening—I didn't understand what happened. Do you know what I mean?

Because people were so upset, and they were kind of talking about it. *And I felt so, like insignificant and stupid, and I felt so sad*, you know, for this guy— because it took me a minute to kind of understand the severity of this and what was happening—I mean, it was my first rotation as a third year; it was probably my first week. And *I was like totally overwhelmed* by the whole thing.

And then I was totally kind of brushed away. And it was like—*it was such a horrific event for the resident*, and watching him go through it, that I felt completely not helpful to him at all. And so, what was starting to be kind of like a great sort of mentoring team, and here we're going to learn a lot of stuff—this event happened, *and I saw him* [the resident] *suffering a lot*.

Because I don't know if he was blamed for it or not, but he didn't want to talk about it, he didn't want to tell me about it, and all those kinds of things that occurred with it. And so, that was challenging, and *I felt, you know, insignificant and not helpful* to do anything. I mean, I wasn't responsible for the orders, but *I felt sort of responsible—*. . . as part of the team. *And very helpless,* as trying to help move things forward. (Elonen, June 19, 2020; italics mine)

In this story, the student-physician was not directly involved in the medical error but felt both responsible and helpless at the same time. The incident weighed on her mind so heavily that she ultimately sought out her chief resident to process it.

Another aspect of medicine that can cause suffering for providers lies in the difficult nature of the work. Physicians are "witnesses to suffering" and being a witness to suffering can cause suffering in the witness (Kahn and Steeves 1994). The *DSM5* defines ongoing exposure to trauma, such as repeated exposure to death or serious injury within the context of one's profession, as a criterion for post-traumatic stress disorder (PTSD). This diagnostic element is particularly applicable to surgeons, intensivists, and emergency room doctors as well as front-line workers such as EMTs who continually witness terrible events (cf. Tangherlini 1998). I asked pediatric oncology surgeon Dr. Corgain about this aspect of doctoring.

> **LG:** Can you talk a little bit about your understandings of the ways in which physicians may suffer as a part of their work?
>
> **DC:** I mean, it should be expected, right? I mean, the nature of what we do is you're entering into suffering, right? Every patient you see has some problem that they're suffering with. And if you're compassionate, you're going to share in that suffering.
>
> And in some cases, what they're suffering through is horrible, you know? Whether it's parents where a child has just been diagnosed with cancer, or a premature baby that's born that has life-threatening anomaly, or a healthy kid that's involved in a trauma that's life-threatening. I mean, *it's horrible suffering that you're recognizing in the world.*
>
> I think for most people, as they go through life you may have one friend or one neighbor that experiences this once. *And the reality of it is, this is what you do every day.*
>
> So, I think there's a part of it that just being in the presence of that suffering, if you have empathy, you're going to suffer also.
>
> And I think that can kind of create a low-grade or medium-grade suffering, just as a part of what you do every day.
>
> Hopefully, within that you have some hope that you're relieving it in some way, either through fixing a problem, or at least being present with people. But even with that, it's fatiguing. (Interview, December 19, 2019)

Dr. Corgain pointed out that most people only endure suffering a few times in their lifetimes, such as the death of a child or other loved one, a debilitating illness, or a life-changing accident. These events are tragic but usually mercifully rare. In contrast, physicians consistently encounter tragedy, illness, and death over and over again in their work, and they are legally and ethically responsible for trying to make such events better or at least lessen their severity. This makes the suffering and death of other people entirely embedded in the work-related duties of physicians, yet very little is done to help physicians and physicians-in-training cope with their own, sometimes very strong, emotional responses (Curtis and Levy 2014).

Some specialties deal with death and suffering on a regular basis. Dr. Massey is a neonatologist whom I interviewed in 2019. She worked in a NICU (neonatal intensive care unit) in Utah and took care of very sick, usually premature babies. Dr. Massey loved her job and found it very gratifying. When I asked her how taking care of sick babies changed her as a person, for example, she responded that it helped her appreciate the miracle of life:

> I think to be at the beginning of life on a regular basis is quite magical. And to see families with a newborn baby struggle, and to see the different things they go through—it gives me a lot of perspective in the rest of my life.
>
> Every minute my children are healthy, they can breathe, they can swallow, they can run, they can—just really basic things are amazing. And it helps me appreciate life in so many ways. That every little thing a baby does is miraculous, you know? (Interview, November 5, 2019)

But working in the NICU also meant being immersed, every day, in the sad fact of very sick or dying babies. I asked Dr. Massey how she learned to cope. She immediately responded, "A lot of tears." She then continued, "Over the years, for me, it's been a variety of things. I think I can usually get through the moment pretty well; I find myself in hallways, just bawling, where no one can see me. I find myself—the next morning, after a baby dies . . . just crying, 'Why? Why do I work in a job where babies die?'" Dr. Massey added that her NICU had improved in terms of helping physicians deal with trauma at work but that this was a recent development: "I have been in this NICU for seventeen years, and in the last five years, we're actually paying more attention to the trauma that doctors and nurses and caretakers experience during the hard times, and when babies die. . . . We are trying to have very specific . . . debriefing[s] . . . more often now. We try to be more rigid about the debriefing, and making sure all the staff has some kind of voice when a baby dies." She stated that the doctors she works with attend their patients' funerals, which also helps them deal with grief.

> We're unusual: we attend the babies' funerals, especially when they've been here for a long time. Because the difference for a newborn is that they've never gone home: we take care of babies who've never been home. And so, this family has not had their child in their own home. Their child has been in our care for their entire life, and we care for the baby when they're not here. And so, we are this child's other family, and it helps give them closure, as well, when they see us at the funerals. . . . Baby funerals are very sad. And it's also another time for me to process that information and be a part of that. (Interview, November 5, 2019)

Memories of particularly difficult or intense cases can stay with physicians for years even if death does not occur. Dr. Corgain recalled:

As an intern—[I had] one particular patient I remember, Charlie, who was a man who had a horrible injury and ended up with severe lung disease as a result. At that point, University of Michigan was really kind of one of the leaders in doing kind of long-term cardiopulmonary bypass, to try to bridge people through this time when their lungs are diseased.

And so, it was called ECMO [extracorporeal membrane oxygenation] when he got sick he was too sick even for that as an investigational thing. And there was a different investigational thing that was kind of on an FDA [Food and Drug Administration] early trial phase, where you put this special device into the big vein in their abdomen, try to give them oxygen that way. And ultimately, that device wasn't approved because it wasn't that successful.

But he was the one patient that survived with it. And so, he was there hundreds and hundreds of days. And it was very complicated. The first months my internship were trying to help him stay alive. And then by the later parts of the internship, it was trying to help Charlie get enough nutrition so that he could get well enough to go home.

So, yeah—so, you have these experiences where it's months and months of you trying to wrestle through these things with patients like that, and then along the way there's these bumps, these horrible life-threatening events that you have to manage. So there's definitely some of those patients that are very clear in your mind, that you know, gosh, twenty-five years later—and I still remember his whole name. (Interview, December 19, 2019)

In this story, the physician worked intensely with the patient for months on end. Dr. Corgain did not say whether or not the patient survived, but the case was intense enough that he remembered it decades afterward.

Physicians are not just passive witnesses to suffering; they actively intervene. This responsibility means that they sometimes must make difficult decisions that result in their own moral injury. One definition of moral injury is "a deep soul wound that pierces a person's identity, sense of morality, and relationship to society" (Silver quoted in Talbot and Dean 2018), which closely overlaps with Cassell's ideas of suffering. A soul wound that "pierces a person's identity" parallels Cassell's notion that suffering entails a threat to personhood and identity, while the pierced sense of morality and relationship to society suggests Cassell's criterion of isolation and meaninglessness. Dr. Corgain talked about some of the grim decisions he made that resulted in his own moral injury and contributed to his own suffering over time.

I think there are other times when you suffer because you may know that there's an ideal thing that can be done, and for whatever practical reason, you can't accomplish it: either you don't have the resources, you're in some other country, some hassle with reimbursement insurance or available facilities, or the distance you are from the facility where you recognize that there's something that could be done that's not done.

So, I think more the social challenges that a particular patient's in . . . those are things, I think, [that] kind of acutely make the suffering worse.

. . . . I volunteer in Kenya. So, we take care of kids there, and we can really do quite a bit there, compared to what is done in a lot of countries. But it's not the same as North America. So, we've got two ventilators for kids, so it means that it's not infrequent that we'll make a decision about what child will be ventilated, and therefore, what child won't get a ventilator. And the natural consequence is that they'll die. So, just that limitation of resources [can cause suffering]. (Interview, December 19, 2019)

Dr. Corgain contributed his time and resources to volunteer in a poor, under-served region of the world, but due to limited resources, he made choices that directly led to saving the lives of some children and the death of others. This moral injury directly contributed to his own personal suffering by engendering feelings of shame, powerlessness, and a threat to core moral identity. This example of moral injury is only one of the many hundreds of traumatic situations physicians may find themselves in over the course of their career. The sadness and grief fade but do not go away. Such experiences are a direct result of their work.

Some of the most extreme working conditions that cause trauma and suffering for physicians are times of national crisis, such as mass shootings or the COVID-19 pandemic. The nation relies on its doctors during these periods but provides little relief or support. Mass shootings, for example, are horrible situations in which multiple people are shot at the same time. Those who do not die instantly need immediate medical care, creating chaotic situations that overwhelm hospitals and staff. Dr. Alejandro Tovar, a surgeon at the University Medical Center of El Paso, had worked thirty hours straight before he was called back into the operating room to operate on the victims of the El Paso mass shooting of August 3, 2019, in which twenty-two people were killed. Fourteen victims needed immediate care, and the hospital cared for a total of thirty. Time was so urgent that the surgeons did not even close the patients' abdomens before moving onto the next victim. The wounds were terrible, and most of the patients required multiple surgeries.[6]

Public discussions about mass shootings usually focus on gun control issues or the victims rather than care providers who attempt to fix the damage. When discussions do focus on doctors, their efforts commonly are described in terms like *lifesaving* and *heroic*, descriptions that play into normative heroic narratives about doctors that arose in the late nineteenth century and coincided with the rise of scientific medicine. The rise of the doctor-as-hero trope followed on the heels of earlier portrayals in the late eighteenth and early nineteenth centuries of the physician as a ghoulish figure. In some of those early novels, physicians were portrayed as unemotional and cruel: they were interested only in the workings of the human body and purposefully inflicted painful or deadly medical procedures on their patients with no sympathy for the suffering that they induced (C. Davis 2020).[7]

Heyward Brock (1991, 285) writes that Henrik Ibsen was the first playwright to treat physicians seriously and the theme of physician-as-hero eventually became a common trope in modern literature, film, comics (Tilley 2018), and television in the twentieth century. Early television programs—such as *Ben Casey* (1961–66), *Marcus Welby, M.D.* (1969–76), and *Dr. Kildare*, which first premiered as a film in 1937—idealized the almost-always-male physician, placed him in a hospital setting, and framed him as heroic: "They usually save lives with ease, mend marriages, reconcile alienated families, give patients the will to live, and continually reassert the primacy of the doctor-patient relationship" (Malsheimer cited in Strauman and Goodier 2011, 32–33).

Communication scholars Elena Strauman and Bethany Goodier (2011, 32) examined television medical drama and wrote that "large and varied audiences have learned much about physicians and what to expect while in their care from television's classroom." Physicians are part of this audience, and such fictional portrayals therefore seep into the lives of real doctors. Medical school students are sometimes told straightforwardly they are heroes: in the late 1990s, for example, I attended a lecture titled something like "You Can Be a Hero" given to medical students at Indiana University medical school in Bloomington. There are also personal pieces published in medical journals and monthly newsletters that draw on heroic ideas with titles like "The Hero in Medicine" (Radetsky 2015) as well as inspirational stories about physicians from impoverished backgrounds who use their medical career to help others (e.g., Yasin 2018). Doctors themselves acknowledge that they sometimes act as heroes or observe others trying to act in this role (Bendjelid 2015). Joseph Campbell's hero cycle has even been applied to the experience of the physician, including the stages of call to adventure, crossing the threshold, trials and wonders, and attainment and return (Rosenzweig 1996).

It is true that physician efforts can be heroic and lifesaving, but normative heroic narratives obscure the pain endured by providers who witness carnage in situations like mass shootings and who are tasked with putting bodies back together. As a reporter for the *New York Times* wrote, once the adrenaline rush dies down, "physicians struggle to live with the horror of what they have experienced." One El Paso physician, Dr. Weber, stated that she and her colleagues were not immune to post-traumatic stress, but there was little organizational support for—or even time to process—what happened.[8] Physicians are expected to pick themselves up from such experiences, dust themselves off, and continue working, in keeping with normative heroic narratives that eschew emotional vulnerability, weakness, and fallibility.

The COVID-19 pandemic brought these issues to the fore. The public became aware of the painful plight of health care workers in the spring of 2020. There was a nationwide shortage of personal protective equipment and physicians, nurses, and other health care and front-line workers began to get sick and die as a result of their work.[9] In some cases it was communicated to providers unequivocally that their own health and safety was of secondary importance. Craig R. Smith, for example, the surgeon-in-chief at New York–Presbyterian Allen Hospital, wrote to staff in an email on March 16, 2020, that as health care workers, they were expected to keep working. "'Sick is relative,' he [Dr. Smith] wrote, adding that workers would not be tested for the virus unless they were 'unequivocally exposed and symptomatic to the point of needing admission to the hospital. That means you come to work. . . . Period.'"[10] At the same time, both the public and the media widely embraced the image of physicians (and other care providers) as heroes with public signage like "Heroes work here" placed in front of hospitals and with military aviation flyovers, such as the one performed by members of 388th Fighter Wing of Hill Airforce Base in Utah on April 30, 2020.

Doctors soldiered on through the pandemic because that they were trained to do so. One New York emergency room doctor named Steven McDonald dryly explained in an op-ed that he dealt with the pandemic because he was already used to being abandoned:

> There has been an abdication of leadership at the highest levels of this crisis that has trickled down to me, a physician in an ER with inadequate personal protections telling oxygen-starved patients to come back when they cannot speak a full sentence or are coughing up more than one tablespoon of blood. These institutions, just like my attendings, are teaching me a lesson through absence: how to manage a pandemic alone. And I am ready because I have been left alone before.
>
> . . . . And although the world should look to its legislators to provide basic income and housing to vulnerable groups, instead it looks to hospitals, to

doctors, to save as many as possible. And we will do our best to sort the living from the dead, because we cannot say no. Because we work in a system that mandates we say yes. Yes to extra shifts, yes to unsafe working conditions, yes to deciding who lives and who dies. This can-do attitude will be the undoing of many of us.

In the meantime, doctors are left alone to sort through our own mental anguish. Which end-of-life conversation will keep me awake at night in a decade? Which face will flash into my consciousness when I'm commuting to work? Essential to sink or swim is acting now and thinking later. (McDonald 2020)

Some physicians committed suicide during the COVID-19 pandemic. One of the most publicized cases occurred in April 2020, when an emergency room physician named Lorna Breen, medical director of the Emergency Department at New York–Presbyterian Allen Hospital in Manhattan, committed suicide at the age of forty-nine. Dr. Breen was overwhelmed by horror and a sense of helplessness as people died before they could be pulled out of ambulances or in the waiting room. She experienced a breakdown even though she had no prior history of mental health issues, and she did not seek help because of the stigma associated with mental illness and needing help that exists in hospital culture among physicians (see discussion later in the chapter). According to one *New York Times* article, Breen was devastated by the sheer number of people she could not save and mortified that she herself needed help during a time when her expertise was most needed. "Lorna kept saying, 'I think everybody knows I'm struggling,'" her sister Jennifer Feist said. "She was so embarrassed."[11] After her death, her family sought more public recognition that medical culture ignores the suffering of physicians by establishing a foundation. "If the culture had been different, that thought [suicide] would have never even occurred to her, which is why I need to change the culture," Ms. Feist said. "We need to change it. Like, as of today." Dr. Breen's father, Dr. Philip Breen, said, "She tried to do her job and it killed her."[12]

Excessively long hours can also be a contributing factor to physician suffering. Most physicians are happy to work very hard; most physician work experiences are not as dramatic as pandemics or mass shootings; and most physicians do not commit suicide. But the organization of physician work, such as the long hours and intense work schedules, leave very little time to process difficult experiences. Dr. Ingram, cervical cancer surgeon, explained this particular point as it manifested during her training:

It just is absolutely exhausting. Literally, those thirty-six-hour shifts where you were pretty much up and having to perform at the top of your game, for you, personally, but more importantly for patients. And then you would still work the next day—there was no off day. And then you'd do it again a day later. And that just rolled month after month after month.

And I think there's an exhaustion element to it, and emotionally you don't have time to regroup when you have seen things that are hard. . . . There's been few times where I felt like gosh, I might pass out; this is overwhelming. . . . And you don't have time to process that too much; you've got to pull it back together and do the job you're supposed to do. And if it's more than just a hiccup like that, it can be hard. And you can get derailed and not have the time to put it back together. (Interview, February 13, 2020)

Such experiences take their toll over time. Some physicians learn to distance themselves emotionally from patients as a survival strategy. Anesthesiologist Dr. Sean McClean explained:

But I think maybe the most important thing, or at least another whole issue that comes along with (that's being dealt with) is you need to be able to distance yourself some from the patients that you're going to be interacting with. Because it sounds—I think maybe from a lay perspective it sounds really cold; but you just can't treat everybody like they're your grandma . . . *or you'll just go nuts.* You just can't—*there's no way to see the suffering and see, you know, families that are losing an eighteen-year-old daughter of cancer and be able to actually function if you don't see that patient as a patient.* And part of seeing them as a patient is breaking them down into organ systems, into tissue pathology, that kind of thing. You just—you know, I think it's really necessary to be able to do that. (Interview, February 24, 2020)

The issue of distancing themselves from patients is important because physicians sometimes are critiqued for not making more personal connections with their patients—for treating them as patients, not people. Yet perhaps cultivating a personal connection can increase physician suffering. One medical student told me that she suffered more when she personally connected with a patient. She explained, "For instance, we had a child come in who had pretty much been dead on the scene but because she was only six years old, they fought really hard to try to bring her back. And so a lot of people were really hurt by that, and I think it's because a lot of people had children around that age or had a sibling or something like that. So if you can make a human connection it really affects you a lot more" (anonymous, interview, April 10, 2012). Dr. Ingram recalled, "One time [there] was this young person in a neurocritical care intensive care unit, that all of a sudden reminded me of my sister. And once I made that connection, I was like, 'Whoa, whoa; OK, this is hard.' And I had to step out" (interview, February 13, 2020). Therefore, in seeking to improve health care, asking physicians to make deeper connections to their patients, such as being more emotionally available, may be difficult for some doctors. The nature of the work does not allow it and may actually increase physician distress as they do their job.

Work also affects physicians' families. Both male and female physicians said that their families suffered. Neonatologist Dr. Steven Frye explained to me that he felt it was important to spend time with the families of his infant patients. The time, however, was at the expense of his own family: "By the majority of people, I'm loved because they see me as their advocate. Parents love me, because I spend time talking to them; I treat them how I want to be treated. I educate them like I would like to be educated, if it was my child. But it means you stay around, sometimes, a long time. The people who suffer from it is often your family" (interview, November 5, 2019). Physicians with young children may miss their early years, as work-life balance is difficult. Dr. Ingram explained:

> It's been hard on my family. And now, I feel like we're in a good place, but obviously (for me) my kids are currently fifteen and seventeen; so, some of those tough years were in their really formative years. And I needed to be there for my patients, and I had to stay late (until seven or eight). And when they were little, they were in bed.
>
> I might not see them. And probably the most crushing thing, before I fig-ured out how to make this work better, is one of my girls when she was little (probably like six), said, "Hey, Mom, can you come visit us some more?" I was like, "Oh my gosh! No. You know I live here, right?" . . .
>
> . . . . So, then I started—when I would go in on the weekend to round, be-cause as people may or may not know, Monday through Friday you take care of patients (if you're a surgeon), or you take care of in-patients in hospitals. Then Saturday and Sunday you go into the hospital to see how they're doing, hopefully move things forward. So, you may not have clinic or surgeries, but you're checking on patients. It's a seven day[s] a week job; it's like two jobs.
>
> So, then I would start getting up (when they were little) I would get up on Saturdays and Sundays at five, so I could get into the hospital, see all the patients, and get home—sometimes put my pajamas back on and act like I'd just been there. And then we'd get up and have pancake breakfast, or whatever—just to trick them. (Interview, February 13, 2020)

Exhaustion may also affect interactions with their families. Dr. Warner observed that he simply did not sleep as well as he used to, making it difficult for him to be present and attentive.

IW: I've found that I don't sleep as well as I used to. I used to be able to sleep anytime, anywhere—it didn't matter. If I had ten minutes, I was asleep. And now, for instance—last night, I got called at one o'clock in the morning and felt like I had to go evaluate this patient. So, I got up, went into the hospital, evaluated them—and fortunately, they didn't need surgery, but I was up.

I went back home and got another phone call as soon as I got into bed. And then I laid there for—I try not to look at the clock, so I don't know how long it was—but I'm going to guess at least an hour (it could have been up to two, maybe an hour and a half). But I just couldn't fall asleep. . . . My mind was racing, I was awake, and I was done [laughs].

We can do great things and wonderful things for people, and it comes at a sacrifice for us and for our families. I think my family, more so than me, have paid a bigger sacrifice, because I'm not there. And when I am there, I may not be there.

LG: You might be asleep.

IW: I might be asleep, or I might be sitting right next to them and just not interested in interacting. (Interview, January 13, 2020)

Despite difficult physical and emotional work conditions, the expectations of doctors by themselves, their patients, and their institutions are extraordinarily high. To paint with a broad brush, doctors have perfectionistic tendencies (Ellison 2017). Patients expect them to be right, and they expect themselves to be right, as their patients' health depends on it. This perfectionism plays on an old idea, originating in the Greek physician Galen, that physicians think of themselves—and are thought of by others—as infallible or even as gods.[13] Galen was the most famous physician of antiquity apart from Hippocrates, and he influenced medical knowledge and learning, particularly the ideas about the circulation system and anatomy, for over 1,300 years (Nutton 2001, 26). Galen also was temperamental, boastful, and egotistical and often came into conflict with other physicians. As the *Spectator* (2017) declared, "If ever there was a doctor with a 'God complex,' it was Galen." After his death, Galen was compared to God by the seventh-century poet George of Pisidia, who called God "the Galen of our souls," implying that Galen was God of the body (Pisidia in Nutton 2001, 27).[14] This perception was reiterated by Voltaire (1694–1778), who wrote that competent physicians partook of the divine: "Men who are occupied in the restoration of health to other men, by the joint exertion of skill and humanity, are above all the great of the earth. They even partake of divinity, since to preserve and renew is almost as noble as to create" (Voltaire 1901). The idea continues today. One modern example is the 1993 film *Malice*, in which a surgeon named Dr. Ed Hill, played by Alec Baldwin, states, "You ask me if I have a God complex. Let me tell you something: I am God" (cited in Dowd 2011). Another modern example is Dr. Strange, the arrogant surgeon created by Marvel comics who values his own views above everyone else's and who, strangely enough, emerged with actual god-like powers due to an accident.

Physicians don't consider themselves to be gods (well, maybe a few do!), but doctors deal with expectations of infallibility, perfection, and omniscience from themselves and others. These high expectations exist whether or not the physician has slept, exercised, recently eaten, or even gone to the bathroom. Orthopedic surgeon Dr. Price explained:

> If you're on-call—some of these calls you get in the middle of the night mean that you have to get up, out of bed, be up all night, and still do your regular job the next day.
>
> So, that's like the really tough thing, is that as a doctor, everybody expects you to be at like 100 percent all the time; and it's like, well if you're also expected to be woken up at—say you get out of bed at midnight, and you're operating at two or three o'clock in the morning—it's like you're probably not going to be 100 percent. And then if you don't get any sleep, like you're not going to be 100 percent the next day.
>
> But the expectation is, is that you know, you be 100 percent, or [that] you be infallible. And that's just the thing that I don't think people can really understand until you've been in that position. . . . I mean, you should give 100 percent of what you have to any patient, you know, irregardless of anything; but I think there's a public expectation for physicians to be 100 percent. I mean, I would never not give somebody my all, But it can be hard. (Interview, November 8, 2019)

No physician is perfect. Mistakes sometimes occur, or doctors are unable to give their best. Sometimes things just don't go well, even if no mistake was made. Medical error obviously occurs, but the expectation is there should be as few as possible. Medical error in particular can be very difficult. Often mistakes are minor and do not result in harm, but sometimes mistakes injure patients. The patient may recover, but he or she may also sustain long-lasting and serious injuries. Today most teaching hospitals address medical error in "morbidity and mortality" rounds. These rounds (conferencing among professionals about particular patients or cases) are specifically designed to formally talk about medical error. The tone of morbidity and mortality rounds differs from hospital to hospital according to its culture. In some teaching hospitals (and likely more so in the past), physicians can be made to feel publicly ashamed for their error and subjected to intense questioning about their decision-making process. Sometimes blame is deflected onto physicians who are lower on the hierarchy, such as residents and interns. As an example, Dr. Elonen described a particularly devastating incident during her training period. A pediatric patient of hers died while she was a resident. The child's medical team later figured out that the child had been dying for some time, but until then, she felt like she was blamed for the child's death, which naturally caused her great pain and distress.

> There was a patient that I had in my pediatric residency, and he was a child that had bad liver disease, and he was essentially dying, he was DNR [do not resuscitate], he was completely yellow. And he had tubes hanging out from him all over the place.
>
> But he was in the hospital for months. And everybody knew this child—I mean, probably years. I mean, he literally was there, and very connected to all the nurses, physical therapists—I mean, people all knew this child, he was just a happy child. But his prognosis was really bad.
>
> And I remember one time—he was my patient, and I was rounding on him and I got my vital signs, and then checked on him: he seemed to be doing OK. I didn't hear about him at all [in] the night. And then we were rounding on him, and he had coded—he like, literally from the time that I had prerounded on him and rounded, he was coded.
>
> And then all of a sudden, everyone's looking at me like, "How come you didn't notice that he was getting so sick? And what happened last night? And da, da, da, da, da." . . .
>
> And I remember when he died—he coded, and he died, and I was like, "Oh, my God, I've completely missed something; I've done something wrong." This was horrible. . . . But I really suffered alone with that.
>
> And I was like, "Oh, my god—I need to talk about this." And again, the amount of disappointment from the entire floor that knew this patient was like, "Who was taking care of this patient, and how did this patient die?" And all this kind of stuff.
>
> And in the end, everyone was like—this was, you know (again), bound to happen; but no one's—you know, you're never ready for it—. . . And it happened, and I never talked about it with an attending, I never processed it with anybody. . . . And finally, I went to the chief resident and said, "I need to talk about this for my own sort of mental health." I was like, "I need someone to kind of help review this with me and make sure that I'm still OK to be a practicing provider"—you know what I mean? . . . It was pretty traumatic for me. (Interview, June 19, 2020)

My spouse also shared a story about a patient who died. In this example, the patient's family, not the medical providers, placed the blame on him and another doctor.

> **WS:** Well, there wasn't really error, but the procedure did not go as planned. The patient had aberrant anatomy, and there was an artery where it usually isn't, and we put a needle through it and he hemorrhaged to death—not because we missed it, but because his tissues wouldn't hold together. So, we tried to sew the artery together, and the surgeon tried to sew it together; and he just fell apart, and he bled to death.
>
> So that family called the resident that did the procedure a murderer and called me a murderer. And it's just hard to hear. I mean, when a patient dies anyway, it's pretty hard, especially if they're youngish (this guy wasn't; he was in his sixties).
>
> But it's just hard to take. So, when you hear that, and there's sort of this anger directed at you—there's just not a lot of resources to manage that in the hospital . . . for the physicians. I don't really think for the nurses either, honestly; I think for nobody. It's just not oriented that way.
>
> **LG:** And how do people deal with it?
>
> **WS:** Well some people burn out and quit. There was a guy my intern year who just snapped. He was found wandering around in the parking lot talking to himself. And they tried to get him through the intern year—actually, he did get through intern year just doing outpatient. And then he (in the second year) he just quit one day: he just left work and never went back. There [also] was a guy that when I was a second-year fellow . . . overdosed and died. (Interview, September 20, 2019)

Some morbidity and mortality rounds discuss medical error in a supportive way so that everyone understands what happened and measures are implemented to ensure that it does not happen again if possible. This seems to be more the trend in teaching hospitals today. Dr. Corgain told me a story about this type of example:

> Yeah, I can distinctly remember one of my coresidents having a technical complication that resulted in a patient's death. And it was with a particular monitoring line that you feed in through the vein; it goes into the artery and the lung. And they use it to measure pressures in critically low patients. And it ruptured that artery of the lung, and [the patient] bled to death.
>
> And it was a huge issue in the hospital, because it was one of the prominent surgeon's patients. And we have a morbidity and mortality conference

where these things are reviewed, and it was pretty clear, but he was dread-
ing going into this, because you were anticipating that this guy would be
crucified.

And I could distinctly remember, because he presented that case. And the
very first thing was the chairman of surgery, who asked him very specifically,
he said, "Well when that happened, did he cough up blood?"

And I thought, "Well that was a really strange question to ask."

And then he just followed up with, "Because when I did this last year, and
this happened, that's what happened."

And it was kind of this immediate sea-change of okay, it's now no longer
you—we're going to talk about how dangerous this device is, and how we all
need to be circumspect about whether we decide to use it, because they're
intrinsically dangerous and even the most experienced person has this
happen.

I still remember thinking, there's a rescue swimmer in the water for that
kid. (Interview, December 19, 2019)

Even with a healthy discussion, however, medical error can cause significant
psychological pain. Physicians may talk to other doctors who have made similar
mistakes but doing so is an individual decision and not an institutionalized
means of support. And just because someone else made a similar error does
not make the error any easier. One physician privately told me that he replayed
a medical error he made in his head every single day for months and thought
about the patient for years afterward. When medical error happens, physicians
ask themselves, What could I have done differently? What can I do next time so
that this does not happen again? As one doctor told me, "I'll never forget this
patient. I'll never forget what happened." Another stated, "Those things haunt
you; they don't go away."

This sense of failure or guilt can be exacerbated by the public. The family
of the patient, who is grieving, may blame the doctor or the medical team,
who are the most visible point of contact, even if no error is made. Dr. Gibbs
explained to me:

> In psychiatry it's also very difficult because we have kids that come in that
> are suicidal, and we try to diagnose them appropriately, and give them
> medications they need, therapy they need; but sometimes they still commit
> suicide. It's just a fact. But then they blame the doctor for maybe not doing
> enough.... I mean that's definitely changed me: just the weight of that
> responsibility, and then maybe the general public not fully understanding the
> nuances that go into all of this. It's just very easy to blame the one who they
> see as like the top of the pecking order, you know what I mean? It's hard.

And we are doing our best to educate people about this. I think that's one of the newer things in the last (maybe) five to ten years, is more and more education, so people have a better understanding of medicine and what really goes into it. (Interview, September 7, 2019)

In the end, doctoring is difficult work. Doctors do their best, and they help many people. But they also witness terrible things over and over again; they frequently are stressed and overworked; and they have little institutional support for the fraught emotional dimensions of their jobs. Although they do their best, sometimes their best is not enough. Dr. Corgain explained:

Because I think that whatever term you want to put on it, I think that phenomena—and it may not just be moral injury—but this reality of doing your best, [and having it] not be good enough. And even doing your best and maybe hurting someone is actually what makes it hard for people to work.

It's probably not the work hours, it's probably not the fact that you didn't get as much recreational time as other people; it's this loss of sense of meaning—or loss of sense of confidence that you're doing a good job and doing the right thing. I think as I talk to people and listen to people, I think those are really the things that weigh people down and take them out. Because there are lots and lots of surgeons that work lots and lots of hours and are happy. (Interview, December 19, 2019)

I asked Dr. Ingram about how she took care of herself in such a difficult field. She pointed to a Gustav Klimt painting on her wall.

It's called *The Tree of Life*. And I put this up here to remind me of that little black bird in the middle of it. It's a beautiful painting, and there's lots of other intrigue in it.

But to me, there's all this beauty, but there's always, at the center of it, this reminder of life is fleeting and there's some darkness here, and there's some loss that's going to happen. And my job is to try and keep that tree growing. But I don't really have total control that that bird is sitting there—that bird that represents death. And that helps me because I don't have all knowing and all capacity to fix things.

So, some of the tragedy of what I see—and I see it weekly and daily; and I've had this recent run of very young women with advanced cancers: twenty-one-year-old with stage four cervical cancer; thirty-eight-year-old, right now, who is dying in the hospital.

And I guess partly the self-care is trying to remind myself constantly that if I can make it better, even in the short-term—either if it's a pain alleviation, or can I

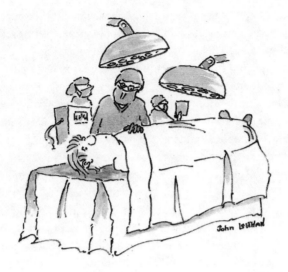

"Just remember, you're not alone -
I'm scared to death, too."

Figure 2.1. Cartoon illustrating physician sharing
inner fears with patient.

extend life for three, six, twelve months? That might be a window where a young mother's kid knows her. And that helps me a lot. (Interview, February 13, 2020)

Structural, Organizational, and Cultural Issues

It was clear from my interviews that doctors sometimes suffered because of work and that it was largely overlooked by physicians themselves and the hospitals. This means that although physician suffering exists, the organizational culture of doctoring stifles it. Role definitions and the structure of the physician-patient relationship contribute to this lack of acknowledgment. It is an old sociological truism that the role of care provider does not allow for sickness. Physicians, nurses, and other health providers care for patients: this is their job. The job is defined by their role. One person, the patient, plays the role of a person who is sick, suffering, and in need of help, and the other person, the physician (or nurse or other health provider), plays the role of the caretaker who provides help. Sociologist Talcott Parsons (1951) examined this relationship in detail, observing that the roles of sick person and physician entailed certain expecta-tions. A sick person is exempt from normal obligations, is not responsible for their own state, is in need of help, and has defined their sickness as undesirable. Physicians are expected to do everything within reason to help the patient, not be upset by the patient's behavior, and manipulate the patient into following recommendations. According to Parson's model, who gets categorized as sick is defined by the role a person takes. Patients, not physicians, are sick and in need of help. To be sick, one must take on the patient role. The physician cannot be sick or suffer because the role does not allow it.

What effects does this role's condition have if one's permanent job is to provide care? It is as though the role overshadows reality. Doctors and nurses obviously get sick and can suffer, but this reality is muffled by their professional role. The object and meaning of work is the sick patient, not themselves. It is therefore very difficult for physicians to admit being sick because doing so recategorizes them as patients. And even if physicians admit to being sick, it remains difficult for them to abandon the role of physician since at any moment they are "on call" and must go back to being a physician. As DeSole, Singer, and Aronson (1969, 301) wrote in an early article addressing this issue, "indeed, he [the physician] is even unable to gain relief from role demands by playing the 'sick role.'"

Another reason it is difficult for physicians to take on the role of patient is that many doctors do not separate their professional role from their individual identity: the link between the two is extremely close. This link is cultivated over the long training period. By the time the period ends, the physician's en-tire sense of self is shaped by work. As Dr. Corgain explained: "I can't imagine, honestly, what I'd would be like if I wasn't a physician. . . . it would be difficult for me to look back, take that twenty-year-old kid in college, and even try to imagine what it would be like at [age] fifty-four without those experiences. I don't know what I'd be without it. So, I think in some sense it's like every bit of who I am is part of that, just shaped by all those experiences" (December 19, 2019). This close link between personhood and physicianhood makes it difficult to take on the role of patient, rendering the existence of physician illness and suffering difficult to acknowledge, even by themselves.

Another reason physician suffering remains hidden is that the occupational culture of doctors emphasizes toughness and the ability to work hard as core values, values that play into normative heroic narratives found in television's medical dramas. The lengthy and intense educational period described in chap-ter 1 trains physicians to keep working at all costs. Hard, even excessive, work is valued: it is a core aspect of a physician's identity. Intern year, residency, and fellowship are characterized by lack of sleep or regular exercise, excessive hours, little leisure time, and no structured mealtimes during the workday, which can last for as long as twenty-eight hours or more if a physician is on call. Physicians therefore learn to deny their own basic physical needs; often there is not even time to go to the bathroom, much less eat or sleep. At the University of Utah, for example, my spouse observed during his residency in the mid-aughts that some residents gave themselves bags of IV fluids when they felt slightly sick so that they could rapidly hydrate themselves in order to keep working.

Compounding this issue is the fact that it is indecorous for physicians to complain about their own problems when they care for people who are presumably in worse condition. As anesthesiologist Dr. Mark York explained in an interview conducted in 2018:

> **MY:** And the other piece of that is that it's very hard for us, and nurses, and PAs [physician's assistants], and all of the healthcare professions. . . . It's very hard for us to complain. Right? I did a liver transplant on Monday night with this lady who, right now, I'm sure, three days later is lying in the ICU in some considerable pain—but she's got a new liver, but she's in pain. . . . Right? It's hard for me to complain about whatever . . . when I'm taking care of people with cancer, and trauma, and you know, they've lost a baby, and all these other things—how can you?
>
> **LG:** You can't say, "I have a cold," if you don't feel good today.
>
> **MY:** Yeah, or even just, "Oh, I had to type for twenty minutes on my computer." But it's very hard to complain . . . in a public forum, when you are taking care of people who have these spectacularly awful situations. We always consider it, "Well it's not that bad." (Interview, September 6, 2018)

The organization of work in many teaching hospitals also contributes to physician suffering because it disincentivizes taking time off for sickness and stigmatizes mental health issues. Taking care of patients is not work that can wait. Sick people do not go away at the end of the day, and dealing with illnesses cannot be put off until tomorrow. Sick patients must always have someone to care for them, and the person who knows the patient best is their primary physician. From a physician's standpoint, it is always best to care for one's own patients. When a physician takes time off from work because they are ill, it means that another physician must cover the sick physician's patients. The covering physician must care for their own patients, any new patients that might come in during that period, and the sick physician's patients, which increases the amount of work that the already-quite-busy covering physician must do. Therefore, taking time off for illness is always at the expense of one's coworkers—and possibly, one's patients—making physicians quite reluctant to take it unless they are demonstrably infectious. This organization of work reinforces the idea that it is unseemly to focus on one's own, supposedly relatively minor needs, when one's job is to take care of patients.

Physician occupational culture also covertly frames physicians who attend to their own needs as being weak, dependent, or needy. Masculine ideas about strength and weakness in relation to sickness—and work more broadly—permeate medical culture. Doctors who do their work well and don't cause work for others may be characterized as "strong," while physicians, residents, and medical students who cannot keep up with the work, who make mistakes that cause additional work for others, and who take too much time off may be seen as "weak." For doctors, being sick, therefore, can be seen by their colleagues as a form of weakness, and doctors about whom their colleagues must worry (meaning they are perceived as not doing their job well) may be called "weak links." My spouse explained this culture as it was reflected in his own residency and fellowship:

> **WS:** Yeah; I think there's sort of this obligation to the team, and a notion like, if you don't show up, you're weak. So, people talk about weakness all the time. So, if someone does a really good job, what you tell them isn't "Awesome job," it's "Strong work."
>
> So, if a resident isn't a good resident, you call him a weak resident. And like when you're coming onto a service that you don't know, you ask the senior residents, "Well who do I [need to watch]?" When I was a fellow, I'd be like, "Well who's the weak residents? Who do I need to worry about?" And that's how you would talk about it.
>
> **LG:** It sounds a little bit like kind of a culture of masculinity.
>
> **WS:** It's hypermasculine. (Sheppard, interview, September 20, 2019)

Attitudes about strength and weakness reflect patriarchal gender norms for men (see Bronner 2005). Medicine historically is white and male dominated. Traditional gender roles for men include strength and the ability to work hard and to endure physical discomfort without complaint, linking notions of what makes a "good" physician to conventional ideas about masculinity. Further, noted scholar Deborah Lupton (2003, 28) writes that illness is feminized because men are reluctant to put their bodies under the control of another person, so a sick man challenges dominant conceptions of masculinity. Evidence of how such ideas become toxic can be found in physicians' own descriptions of their burnout. One physician recalled the kinds of questions he asked himself after he burned out: "Was I too weak? Did I not have enough for-titude, endurance, or grit? *With those thoughts of weakness came feelings of shame*" (Tolpin 2018, italics mine). The physician's description of feelings of shame leads directly back to Cassell's holistic description of suffering.

Medicine exploits traditional roles for women as well. Traditional gender roles for women, particularly mothers, include self-sacrifice and taking care of others at any expense. Medicine today includes both men and women in approximately equal numbers, and so it appears that the occupational culture draws on both types of traditional gender ideologies to create a context in which male and female physicians continually put hard work above their own needs and in which sickness for a physician is stigmatized. This attitude, al-though changing, continues in the twenty-first century. One medical student explained: "I guess one thing I was unaware of . . . [is] that a lot of physicians are humiliated—maybe that's not the right word—but feel like they need to be tough and upstanding, and don't really let themselves, you know, realize that this is really affecting me [i.e., the physician] too—. . . And I need to take care of myself, too" (anonymous, interview, March 21, 2012).

The biggest stigmas for physicians are mental health issues. This is partly due to the occupational culture of denial and its tendency toward perfectionism. Physician therapist Wayne Sotile (2019, 524) notes that "too often, physicians are encouraged to adhere to a code of stoicism, self-denial, and isolation when facing psychosocial pain" and such attitudes create barriers to wellness and seeking help (Duran 2019; Gold, Sen, and Schwenk 2013). The documentary *Struggling in Silence* actively strives to overcome stigma surrounding depression by emphasizing that depression is "real" (that is, based in neurobiology), and it repeatedly emphasizes the effectiveness of medications like antidepressants in order to encourage physicians to seek help.

This cultural stigma is reinforced by structural barriers. Physicians who admit to depression, addiction, or other mental health issues face professional consequences. Physicians are required to disclose mental health issues to li-censing boards and their health care institutions. If they take antidepressants, for example, they are required to disclose that fact. Such disclosures can lead to censure, meaning that they may have their medical license restricted or re-voked, and they can be fired. Mental health issues also go on their permanent record as a kind of black mark. These structural barriers exacerbate the prob-lem, since physicians experiencing mental health issues may hide the fact that they are in distress. The wife of one physician who committed suicide stated in an interview that the health care setting in which her husband worked cre-ated "the perfect storm and a bad environment for mental health" (quoted in

Hoffman and Kunzmann February 5, 2018). Overall then, the occupational culture of physicians downplays their own needs and health issues in the name of patient care, an orientation that ultimately contributes to a culture in which physicians suffer in silence.

It is also true, however, that such attitudes are changing. Early to mid-twentieth-century media representations of doctors portrayed them as heroes, but recent ones portray more complex—albeit still heroic—characters encountering ethically difficult dilemmas (Tilley 2018). One example of a more complex character from the 1990s is Dr. House from *House M.D.* Dr. House was brilliant medically and resolutely scientifically rational but also plagued by personal problems. In medicine, too, there has been a growing interest in physician health and wellness. One therapist who counseled physicians for over forty years wrote that "collectively, we are ending the conspiracy of silence about physician suffering and ill-being that has pervaded our medical culture historically" (Sotile 2019, 524). Recent examples in the medical field include an emphasis on increasing physician resilience, as well as building awareness of and destigmatizing mental health issues (e.g., the work being done by the organization set up by Dr. Lorna Breen's family, the Heroes' Foundation). Humanities perspectives also have been promoted and utilized by faculty at medical schools. One program is Dr. Rita Charron's (1986) narrative medicine program, initiated at Columbia University, which encourages medical students to write about their experiences. One clinic in Cleveland established a "lavender code" in which a support team provides a holistic rapid response to providers during times of crisis.[15] Physicians also have been encouraged to do self-care by increasing activities such as yoga and meditation.

Such efforts are encouraging, although few directly target underlying systemic issues. It is possible for culture to change, but it is slow and difficult. Reform should acknowledge that the heroic narrative is a problematic, culture-wide occupational issue. Dr. Atul Gawande commented that while both the public and physicians would like to see doctors as heroes, an idea that relies on a self-sufficient individual acting alone, modern medicine is actually team-based. He writes, "We've celebrated cowboys, but what we need is more pit crews" (in Morse 2010, 60). He adds, "The stories we doctors tell ourselves about what it means to be great are very important to who we are, but they create a cognitive dissonance. We like to imagine we can be infallible and be that heroic healer. But the fact is, it's teams and, often, great organizations that make for great care, not just individuals. So we need to change these stories we tell ourselves and reshape the discussion" (61). Gawande's point is that medical narratives should be more collective, but he doesn't critique the heroic narrative itself, illustrating how embedded it is in medical culture. Heroic ideals make great novels and television drama, but they set actual physicians up for failure by placing them on a pedestal, leaving little narrative breathing room for doctors to be ordinary mortals who make mistakes, get tired, and cannot always save the day. Such unrealistic, idealized beliefs are toxic for real, on-the-ground working people.

In conclusion, suffering is embedded in medicine. Most physicians understand suffering clinically as the object of work: the purpose of work is to relieve patient suffering if possible. But doctoring has epistemological implications. Doctors witness suffering, and they are tasked with relieving it. They can suffer themselves because the work is difficult and the stakes are high, because of the limitations of medical and social systems, and because of the choices they make. The organization of medical work, including the nature of education, training, and practice, can further compound suffering. Finally, the ethos of medicine can perpetuate physician suffering through an informal code of perfectionism, stoicism, silence, and stigma around illness, a code that is reinforced by institutionalized structural barriers that deter doctors from seeking help. Suffering therefore is both a clinical and a cultural reality, one that remains underexamined. It constitutes the deep context for the humor and laughter of the medical carnivalesque, which is explored and outlined in the rest of this book.

Notes

1. One reason for this high rate may be that due to their extensive knowledge of anatomy, physicians are simply better at successfully killing themselves than other people. See Glaser 2015.

2. It is difficult to obtain completely reliable data about physician suicide for a number of reasons, one of which is that sometimes the cause of death is not actually listed as suicide.

3. I am grateful to Dr. Corgain for pointing me to this term.

4. The definition of trauma and PTSD was significantly revised between the *DSM4* and the *DSM5*. The *DSM5* states that PTSD is not an anxiety-related disorder but rather a "Trauma and Stressor-Related Disorder," which meant that trauma itself became a new diagnostic category. The definition of trauma also narrowed in the *DSM5*. The *DSM5* definition of trauma required "actual or threatened death, serious injury, or sexual violence" (Pai, Suris, and North 2017, 271). Stressful events not involving an immediate threat to life or physical injury such as psychosocial stressors (e.g., divorce or job loss) are not considered trauma in this definition. Trauma and stressor-related disorders, like PTSD,

require exposure to trauma as a precondition. The types of qualifying exposures include direct personal exposure, the witnessing of trauma to others, indirect exposure through trauma experience of a family member or other close associate, and repeated or extreme exposure to aversive details of a traumatic event, which applies to workers as part of their professional responsibilities.

5. *Oxford English Dictionary*, s.v. "suffering," last modified September 2023.

6. Gina Kolata, "Surgeons Labored to Save the Wounded in El Paso Mass Shooting," *New York Times*, August 9, 2019.

7. I am grateful to my colleague Joyce Kinkead for pointing me to this material.

8. Kolata, "Surgeons Labored."

9. Michael Schwirtz, "Nurses Die, Doctors Fall Sick and Panic Rises on Virus Front Lines," *New York Times*, March 30, 2020. See also Michael Rothfeld, Jesse Drucker, and William K. Rashbaum, "The Heartbreaking Last Texts of a Hospital Worker on the Front Lines," *New York Times*, April 15, 2020.

10. Schwirtz, "Nurses Die."

11. Corina Knoll, Ali Watkins, and Michael Rothfeld, "'I Couldn't Do Anything': The Virus and an E.R Doctor's Suicide," *New York Times*, July 11, 2020.

12. Ali Watkins, Michael Rothfeld, William K. Rashbaum, and Brian M. Rosenthal, "Top E.R. Doctor Who Treated Virus Patients Dies by Suicide," *New York Times*, April 27, 2020.

13. Galen was born in AD 129 and died sometime between AD 216 and AD 217. Galen was controversial because his methods conflated the roles of physician and deity. He introduced the prognosis, for example, in which the physician predicted outcomes for the patient and the disease rather than relying on mysticism and divination. This idea was so controversial that Galen was threatened with assassination (Nutton 2001).

14. Physicians also were thought to have God complexes because they were agnostic or atheistic. Galen, for example, believed in pre-Christian gods but thought that cures were scientifically explainable, and he apparently was vocal about his doubts about the soul. Galen therefore was labeled as a nonbeliever by early Christians, and certainly many early physicians held pagan sympathies well into the sixth century (Nutton 2001, 21–25). The reference to Pisidia is Pisidia's *Hexaemeron*, lines 1388–9, 1544.

15. "Code Lavender: Offering Emotional Support through Holistic Rapid Response," *Consult QD*, November 22, 2016.

3

Death, Life, and Other Absurdities

Comic and absurd representations of death are a pervasive theme in ancient representations of the carnivalesque, especially in juxtaposition to life. One image, for example, is a highly ambivalent image of the pregnant, laughing crone, which conflates old age with fertility. The ancient crone is presumably close to death, well past her child-bearing years, while her pregnant belly represents new life and good health. Dismemberment also is common. There are descriptions in Rabelais's writings in which bodies are torn apart in war or scenes in which a character is beaten to death, and these scenes often are described in a lively manner, accompanied by laughter. The well-known scene of the catchpole is an example. A character called a "catchpole," whose job it is to receive a thrashing, is merrily beaten by Friar John. Once the beating is done, however, the catchpole—who has seemingly died—jumps up again in order to receive another beating. Such scenes are ambivalent. They illustrate the interconnectedness of death and life, and they represent victory over the grave by transforming terror into something comic. The beatings, dismemberment, death, and laughter represent the death of the old world and the birth of the new, a pervasive, encompassing idea.

Comic and absurd references to death and dismemberment also exist in medical contexts. One source is *Gomerpedia*, an online satirical encyclopedia. Written by doctors for doctors, it contains parodic entries of medical terms and terminology. The entry for death, for example, states that "death is defined by the cessation of all biological functions and is typically considered a suboptimal outcome. Patients often state their preference for ongoing life as opposed to death." The entry also states that while it can be challenging

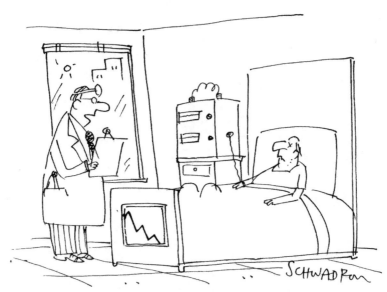

"THE MONITORS ALL SHOW THAT YOU'RE DEAD... BUT to BE SURE, WE'LL NEED to RUN SOME MORE TESTS."

Figure 3.1. Cartoon commenting on unnecessary medical tests.

to elicit symptoms in a patient who has suffered death, "Vital signs can be very telling in a patient with death: temperature is room temperature or less, blood pressure is 0, heart rate is 0, respiratory rate is 0, and oxygen saturation is 0%. Physical exam can be very challenging due to the patient's lack of participation."[1]

The entry is funny not because someone has died but because it transforms something natural and obvious (death, a dead person) into something complicated and medicalized that needs to be diagnosed and verified by a physician. The "signs" of death (0 blood pressure, 0 heart rate, etc.) are absurd because they mimic medical signs but are not signs at all; medical expertise, therefore, is totally unnecessary. The entry then, does not poke fun at death per se but at the medical response to it. This target—the institutionalized, official, medicalized response to death—underlies much death-related folklore in medicine (fig. 3.1). Such folklore is carnivalesque because it highlights comic or absurd aspects of death and the dissected body, ridicules official, elite organizational stances, and is fundamentally ambivalent. It constitutes an important aspect of the medical carnivalesque.

The Denial of Death

Doctors spend their entire professional careers haunted by the specter of death. Cultural critic Lawrence Samuel (2013, x) writes that "science and medicine are of course at the heart of death, so much so that some have argued that their unstated purpose all along has been to solve the 'problem' of dying." The cadaver dissected in gross anatomy lab is considered medical students' "first patient" (Duncan 2018), and as students move through medical school and postgraduate training, they become progressively more responsible for their patients' health. If one goal of medicine is to promote health and healing, then conversely another goal is to stave off sickness and death as long as reasonably possible. Certainly one would be considered a poor physician if one's patients all died. Even primary care physicians, who do not directly care for the critically ill, look for signs of illness and disease. Other occupations may be immersed in death in various ways (funeral directors and priests for example) but few other professions directly seek to keep death at bay.

Physicians also work within a Western European cultural framework that denies death and has done so for nearly two hundred years. Historian Arnold Toynbee (1968, 131) famously observed that "death is 'un-American'" and contradicts the American way of life. Toynbee's observation is supported by others, such as the great poet Octavio Paz (1961, 57) who observed that "the word death is not pronounced in New York, in Paris, in London, because it burns the lips," while Samuel (2013, xi) writes that "if there is one single idea that summarizes the literature devoted to death and dying in America over the last half century or so, it is denial." Death is a "taboo topic," surpassing even sex as something one does not talk about in polite company (Samuel 2013, 80).

This aversion to death developed nationally in the late nineteenth and early twentieth centuries, when social and cultural attitudes rapidly shifted. Until the Civil War, people encountered death regularly in their daily lives. People died at home in the care of family. Women prepared the body for burial, an extension of their traditional role of caring for the sick. Shrouding women specialized in preparing bodies for funerals, and helping a bereaved family was a neighborly duty (Rundblad 1995). Wakes and funerals were held at home.

By the turn of the twentieth century, however, advances in science and medicine, an increased abundance of food and material goods, an ever-increasing sense of individualism, faith in rationality and progress, increasing secularism, the rise of hospitals, and growth of the funerary industry all contributed to distance death from most Americans, culminating in what the historian Philippe Ariès (1975, 1981) called death "denied" by the mid-twentieth century. Burial scholar Suzanne Kelly (2012, 38–39) states that "it is ... no secret that over the course of the last century that stark material reality of death—the corpse— has become increasingly hidden from our sight." Embalming, for example, became the preferred way of preparing the body. It was thought (falsely) that decaying bodies spread disease. Embalming was considered more sanitary than allowing the body to decay naturally (Kelly 2012). Embalming could not be accomplished at home since it involved injecting the body with toxic chemicals (arsenic in the nineteenth century and formaldehyde in the twentieth), and so the task of caring for the dead shifted from women at home to men in professional and sanitized environments such as funeral parlors, marking the institutional- ization of death care. The result was that fewer laypeople interacted with the dead in their ordinary lives, and by the 1950s, home funerals were uncommon.

Other factors also contributed to the cultural denial of death in the twen- tieth century. Mortuaries developed practices designed to hide death, such as beautifying the body with makeup and arranging it in lifelike positions. Specialized caskets prevented decay. British author Jessica Mitford's classic exposé of the funeral industry *The American Way of Death* (1963) targeted these expensive burial practices with biting criticism. The introduction of cadaver gurneys in hospitals also masked death in institutions, and overall such practices "contribute[d] to the deep distance between the living and the dead" (Kelly 2012, 39). There also was a concomitant shift in language toward euphemistic terms surrounding death: undertakers became morticians, cof- fins became caskets, and graveyards became more commonly called cemeter- ies. Americans avoided speaking about death directly. Phrases such as "kick the bucket," "meet their maker," "give up the ghost," "pass away," "go to their reward," "expire," or "pass on" helped people avoid the word "dead" in conver- sation. Literary scholar Louise Pound (1936, 195) famously observed this trend and collected various euphemisms for death, the dead, and dying in an article published in 1936, noting cheekily, "It appears, in fact, that one of mankind's gravest problems is to avoid a straightforward mention of dying or burial."

Hospitals and organized medicine played a prominent role in the denial of death by medicalizing and rationalizing it. The term "to rationalize" means to make more efficient and to control outcomes through the implementation of technocratic decisions and practices, which are often enacted through large bureaucracies. Rationalization is a common feature of modern life, and it is linked to characteristics such as power, surveillance, and control (Scott 1998). The medical rationalization of death during the twentieth century meant that death was masked as disease and that the dying were moved to hospitals, where death became a medical issue and the dying were safely hidden from public view (Ariès 1981, 564–66). Sickness and old age also were moved to institutions, such as nursing homes and care facilities.

Medical language contributed to the denial of death, not only mirroring the larger cultural trend of avoidance through euphemisms, but also helping create it (Peterson 1998). This manner of speaking was observed early in the twentieth century: "The word 'death' is seldom heard in hospital wards" (Barkley 1927, 314). Instead, personnel in the 1920s might have said "to cease breathing" or "to expire." Death was considered such a sad and painful topic that physicians in the mid-twentieth century did not tell patients they were dying. Instead they told the family, whom, according to Ariès, then pretended like nothing was happening in order to not upset the patient. Long periods of mourning were discouraged, as the bereaved were supposed to grieve quietly and quickly move on. The result was that by the mid-twentieth century "the hospital [became] the place of the solitary death" (Ariès 1981, 571). It was private and isolating for both the dying and mourners. Ariès characterized this style of death as "invisible": dying was constructed to be quiet, unobtrusive, and convenient to the living.

Attitudes toward death have shifted since the mid-twentieth century. Newer perspectives reimagine death as a natural part of life and seek to demystify and demedicalize death and dying through strategies such as hospice care, while right-to-die and death with dignity movements strive to empower and dig-nify dying people.[2] The American Medical Association followed these shifts, decreeing in the 1980s that patients had the right to know they were dying. Today about 90 percent of physicians tell their patients they are dying, as com-pared to only about 10 percent in the 1970s (Samuel 2013, xv). The subject of death and dying—how to talk about it with patients, how to process one's own emotions in response to patient death—also recently has been included in some medical school curricula, and conversations about how to ethically approach issues of death and dying are ongoing among medical professionals.

Historical attitudes toward death linger, however, as medicine continues to attempt to rationalize and control it. In the midcentury, death was considered a defeat and everything was done to avoid it; today, that attitude has lessened but has not been erased. Contemporary medical expressions continue to veil the fact that someone died, such as the phrase to "have a negative patient out-come" (Burson-Tolpin 1989, 287). Another linguistic strategy uses passive or indirect descriptions, as in a patient who "fails to live." The use of the passive voice especially has long been considered a way to avoid areas that are pain-ful for physicians. It is impossible to generalize about individual beliefs and attitudes, but many doctors feel that it is their responsibility to stave off death, a belief encouraged by the wider culture that still views death in a negative light. Advances in technology and the desire of physicians and patients to use technology contribute to ongoing attempts at rationalization. And as physicians are responsible for their patients' health, death for physicians can be seen as an enemy and a source of anxiety, guilt, and personal failure (McCrary and Christensen 1993). The death of a patient may also contribute to a physician's own suffering (see chapter 2).

Death-related folklore in medicine therefore exists within a complicated series of nesting fields. Physicians seek to keep sickness and death at bay, and they do so as experts working within an institutionalized context that rationalizes biological processes. This rationalization historically has contributed to a larger cultural denial that made death a taboo topic. Humor often arises around areas of taboo, and so it is no surprise that death-related humor exists. As processes of life and death have become medicalized and rationalized in the modern era, a carnivalesque perspective has emerged that subverts such official, institutionalized stances.

Gross Anatomy

Gross anatomy is a required laboratory class usually taken during the first year of medical school. It is here that students confront in intimate ways the stark materiality of death that American culture works hard to avoid. Harvard medical student and NPR commentator Joe Wright (2005) reflects, "To dissect a cadaver is to immerse oneself in the immutable fact of death," yet gross anatomy may be the first time a student sees a cadaver up close. As one student observed in a letter she wrote to her cadaver, "Before you, I had never seen a corpse, and I had only once confronted death, when I visited my great-grandmother near the end of her life" (Low 2010).

Death-related folklore first emerges in gross anatomy lab, although pre-med college students may encounter it earlier (Hafferty 1988, 349). The first and easiest joke is that gross anatomy is called "gross" for a reason. At some schools, such as at the University of Maryland–Baltimore, the class quickly is nicknamed "the gross lab" (Block 2004a). This term is known across the country. I asked one medical student why humor in the gross anatomy lab exists. They explained, "I mean, yeah—like in anatomy lab, like there's always just like weird humor, because you're literally dealing with someone's—that was someone's wife, or mom, or grandma, and you're holding their heart, and you don't know them. . . . So, it's a very awkward, existential place to be: in somebody's body that you don't know" (anonymous, interview, March 21, 2012).

The student's comment that the class puts people in "awkward, existential places" speaks to the boundaries that are crossed and transgressions that occur with respect to the body in gross anatomy. As one psychiatrist commented in the documentary *The First Patient*, medical students have been authorized to do things in gross anatomy that no one else is authorized to do. Students are highly aware of the social and cultural taboos they are violating. One student pointed out in a written reflection, "I had peeled the skin off of a human body. I had just done something that would have been viewed as insane had it not taken place in an academic context" (Reifler 1996, 189). Death-related folklore mediates these violations.

Students encounter their donor on the first day of lab, which usually is a large room and quite cold. The number of cadavers depends on the class size. Each cadaver is placed on a metal table, covered with a plastic sheet, and situated below an exhaust hood, which vents the overpowering smell of formalin, a preservative. A constant current of cool air blows. Students work on their donors in groups of three to six throughout the semester/year (depending on the school and availability of cadavers) and come to know their cadaver intimately. In gross lab students spend hours upon hours with "their" cadaver, cutting skin, melting fat, sawing bones, examining nerves. Dissected body parts, connective tissue, bits of skin and fat may be kept in a covered biohazard bucket under the dissection table until the end of the semester/year, as this material was when I visited the gross anatomy lab at Indiana University–Bloomington in 1999.

The smell of formalin, which is used to preserve the bodies and may be referred to as "cadaver juice," saturates the lab. The smell is overpowering and difficult to remove from clothing and hair, and so one of the earliest experiences for medical students is that they immediately start smelling like their cadaver. I used to joke with my partner after he returned from lab that he "smelled like death," and Dr. Warner, recalling his experiences in anatomy lab recalled, "But then the smell. The formaldehyde stays with you—it does not go away" (Interview, January 13, 2020). When NPR's Melissa Block asked medical students at the University of Maryland how much of the gross lab they took home with them, one student answered, "I think all you really need to do is smell our hands right now to know exactly how much this follows us. As soon as I get home, especially like on Fridays, which is when I see my girlfriend. The first thing she makes me do is hit the shower with as much scented stuff as possible. It's pretty intense" (Block 2004b). And one student even wrote reflectively in a letter to her cadaver, "The funny thing about working with your body is that I've become a little embalmed myself. No matter how long I scrub my arms with exfoliating grapefruit scrub, the smell of embalming fluid never seems to go away" (Low 2010).

The term *anatomy* comes from the Greek word *anatemnein* and the Latin word *anatomia*, meaning to cut up into parts, making the study of anatomy and dissection almost synonymous (Moxham and Plaisant 2014, 220). Forms of human dissection have existed since ancient times, but the act historically has been fraught with religious and moral taboos, beliefs, and circumscribed practices surrounding corpses and treatment of the dead. The Greek physician Hippocrates refused to dissect, while Aristotle and Galen dissected mostly animals. Dissections within the Roman Empire were prohibited until the Middle Ages; the first formal dissection in Europe was held at the University of Bologna in Italy in 1156.[3] One dissection was allowed every five years after 1240 per an edict from Holy Roman emperor Frederick II, but in general, "before the Renaissance a tussle existed between anatomists who wished for research and teaching purposes to undertake human dissection and the authorities, both religious and secular, who wished to prohibit dissection" (Moxham and Plaisant 2014, 226).

The study of anatomy became important during the early modern period although dissection remained controversial, viewed as immoral by the church and society in general. The University of Bologna approved dissection as a means of teaching anatomy in 1405 and built a famous, elaborate dissecting theater with elevated seating from which viewers could better observe the proceedings; others followed (see figure 3.2 for an example of an anatomy theater).[4] Fine artists such as Michelangelo (1475–1564) and Leonardo da Vinci (1452–1519) studied anatomy to better represent the human form, although da Vinci's anatomical illustrations went unpublished for many years.

The most famous anatomist of the period was Andreas Vesalius, born in 1514, and known as the father of modern anatomy. Vesalius studied first at the University of Louvain in Belgium and then at the University of Paris, where he became famous for conducting his own dissections rather than merely overseeing them. After he obtained his medical degree, he was granted the title of professor of surgery at the University of Padua. He became the first anatomist to directly contradict the received wisdom of Galen and Avicenna (see note 2). At the time, few anatomists recorded their own observations because the nature of knowledge construction meant repeating traditionally received knowledge rather than adding one's own ideas. They also did not draw or record their observations because pictures were taboo; anatomical manuscripts were text-based only. Vesalius produced his own illustrations and helped the university "generate knowledge from experience and observation and not on scholastic

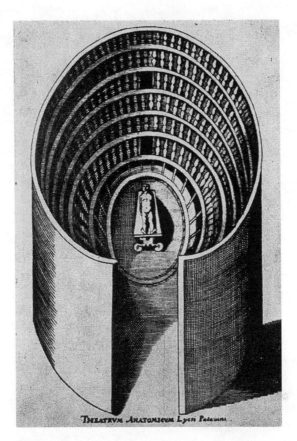

Figure 3.2. Padua anatomy theater, 1654. Illustrator unknown.

principles that merely relied upon reading and reinterpreting existing texts" (Moxham and Plaisant 2014, 229).

Procurement of corpses was always problematic. The only corpses made formally available for dissection until the early nineteenth century were those of condemned criminals and even those only rarely. In France, for example, after 1376 at the University of Montpellier, the "body of an executed criminal was available for dissection annually," linking the means of procuring a corpse directly to the justice system and making dissection a punishment (Moxham and Plaisant 2014, 226). The Murder Act of 1751 in Great Britain specified that people executed for murder would not be given a burial and instead their bodies were either to be gibbeted or made available for public dissection.

As medical knowledge expanded in the eighteenth century the demand for corpses led to an increase in the practice of bodysnatching. Groups of men in the UK called "resurrectionists" robbed graves. The corpses were sold to physicians and anatomists at market price.[5] The most famous scandal during this period occurred in Edinburgh, Scotland, where a resurrectionist named William Burke and his cohorts not only robbed graves but also murdered people and sold their bodies to a physician named Dr. Robert Knox. The murders were eventually discovered, Burke was executed, and his body dissected publicly as punishment. The scandal led to the Anatomy Act of 1832, which more formally regulated bodies for dissection by giving anatomists access to the unclaimed corpses of people who died in prisons or poorhouses.[6]

The social, cultural, and institutional taboos surrounding the dissection of corpses have lessened significantly over time. People today willingly donate their bodies to science. Bodies mostly are procured through donations and bureaucratic processes rather than through the prison system or poorhouses.[7] No one is dissected publicly as punishment. The history of dissection therefore is an excellent example of how medicine has rationalized the practice. Over time and using formalized procedures, laws, bureaucracies, and attitudes of detachment, dissection has been successfully reframed as an impersonal, scientific enterprise designed to further medical education and therefore, presumably, the common good.

But traditional feelings, beliefs, and responses to death, corpses, and anatomization remain for many students, at least initially. Gross anatomy differs from other classes that first-year medical students take such as microbiology or pharmacology for the obvious reason that students must completely dissect an entire human body to pass the class, including the most intimate parts such as the face, hands, and genitalia. Students must overcome feelings of nausea, disgust, revulsion, and horror as the successful dissection of a human cadaver is crucial to the construction of a medical identity. The body of literature that exists on students' responses to human dissection indicates that some students find gross anatomy distressing or unnerving (though certainly not all; many students enjoy it). Gross anatomy can generate strong emotional responses for some students, including nightmares, death anxiety, and detachment, although these responses usually decrease as the course progresses. A minority of students even experience "dissection trauma" (Hancock et al. 2004) or symptoms similar to post-traumatic stress disorder (Finkelstein and Mathers 1990).

Studies also conclude that "the use of coping mechanisms is an important medical competency mediated by the dissection course" (Tseng and Lin 2016, 266). In addition to learning about the human body, a latent function of gross anatomy class is to teach students to control their emotions and responses in the name of professionalization (Segal 1988). Medical professionalization means the ability to view and handle the body in a calm and rational manner, without reacting emotionally, such as with horror, disgust, or lust. Not only has medicine rationalized death, the corpse, and anatomization, but the class rationalizes the students themselves by socializing them into viewing the human body through a technocratic perspective. As anthropologist Daniel Segal (1988) notes, the body is constructed as an object and the physician's authority is reified as an agent who handles the body of others in a professional manner.

Death-related folklore and carnivalesque laughter emerge in contradistinction to this professionalized and technocratic response to death and anatomization. Katharine Young (1997, 127) concluded as much after she was warned by a chief pathologist that she should not give way to "unseemly merriment" as she was escorted into a morgue. She writes that not only is corpse-related humor evidence of metaphysical unease about the ontological status of the dead body but that the laughter it evokes is carnivalesque as it threatens the "aristocracy" of medical discourse (128).

One of the most important aristocratic values in the gross lab from the viewpoint of the institution, for example, is to treat the cadaver with the utmost respect. This is the way all gross anatomy labs officially are conducted. The cadaver formally is referred to as "the donor" and medical students use this term throughout the year. Donors are anonymous; students may not know the donor's name or birth date or why or how they died, although the cause of death, such as cancer, may become obvious once dissection begins. Such anonymity is functional, as it is easier to dissect an anonymous medical specimen than a person with a history and personality. It is one aspect of the larger process of the medical rationalization of death, which provides the framing through which dissection occurs.

Anatomy instructors emphasize that the donor is a teacher from which students learn. They stress that the donor has given a precious gift to the students and that the students are privileged to learn from it, a perspective that students internalize. As one student I interviewed emphasized: "I took the anatomy lab and our body donors very, very seriously, and really wanted to show our body the most respect that we could. So, I feel like I am probably in the upper percent of the class that would have like a problem with . . . the joking" (anonymous, interview, March 21, 2012). Students featured in the documentary *The First Patient* (2018) also emphasized the preciousness, importance, and sacrifice of the donor. Many medical schools emphasize the importance of the donor by holding remembrance ceremonies, funerals, and in some cases, even having the donor's family meet the students (although these practices do reveal the donor's identity). Such ceremonies reinforce the officialness and seriousness of the donation and the task at hand.

At the same time, however, official dictates of how students are supposed to feel and act do not fully address anxieties, apprehensions, and fears students may have regarding death and corpses, or the transgressive nature of dissection itself. The corpse is what medical sociologist Frederic Hafferty (1991) refers to as an ambivalent referent. It is both a human being and a learning tool that students are supposed to handle with professionalism and detached concern. It also is a body wrapped in ancient social and cultural taboo, which the students violate. The students therefore find themselves in contradictory positions. Anthropologist Mary Douglas (1968) explains that a joke consists of an incongruity in the social situation, which then requires a humorous utterance to express it. Similarly, death-related folklore mediates the students' paradoxical stances, targeting official responses as well as acknowledging the serious boundaries students cross as they perform their work.

One of the earliest and most traditional ways that students resist institutionalized values is by giving the donor a name or a nickname. This naming tradition dates at least to the nineteenth century and according to one survey published in 2013, 67.8 percent of medical students continue to name their cadaver (Williams et al. 2014). The types of names given to donors vary widely. Sometimes the donor's name/nickname is a real name such as "Joe." One student I interviewed said his group had nicknamed their donor "Fred," because they found Fred to be a very average-sounding name. Other examples are names that sound like the names of older people, such as "Agnes" or "Herman" (Wright 2005), presumably because the donors were old. Students I talked to named their donors "Sally" or "Winnie" or "Artie" (short for Arthur) simply because the donors looked like a Sally or Winnie or Artie. The fact that they were dead but "looked like" a particular name was the crux of the humor.

Some donor names referenced the physical features of the donor or alluded to popular culture. One interviewee said that their group named their donor "Julia" because the donor's fingernails were painted red. The reference was to the sex worker Julia Roberts played in the 1990 movie *Pretty Woman*. Another student told me his group called their donor "the Green Man" and the "Green Lantern" because the cadaver was mysteriously green, while a third group named their donor Ron after the porn star Ron Jeremy, since the donor had died of congestive heart failure, resulting in a large and swollen penis (Gabbert 2020). Other examples based on physical characteristics included "Frank the Tank" because the donor was a physically large person; "Melanie," named for the fact that the donor had moles and presumably, melanoma; and "Tough Old Broad" based on the number of scars on the cadaver (Williams et al. 2014, 173).

Other types of names are clever puns or plays on words: as one female student told NPR's Melissa Block, "We've picked out a name. If it's a boy, it's Reggie Mortis, if it's a girl, it's Regina Mortis" (Block 2004a), while in a similar vein, "Abra-Cadaver" was a name passed on to me by an anonymous informant from the University of Utah (anonymous, interview, September 26, 2019). Yet another interviewee named their cadaver Justin because of the small penis (*ba-dum-tss!*), while Dr. Brian Goldman (2014, 286) recounts a student who named his donor Ernest, as in "I'm working in dead earnest."

Not all students name their bodies. Many students continue to refer to their cadaver as "the donor" out of a sincere attempt to maintain the official atmosphere of respect. Some schools, such as Tulane University School of Medicine, specifically request students not name their donors since the donors already had a name in life (anonymous, personal communication, September 5, 2019). But naming a donor is not de facto disrespectful, even if the name is playful or off-color. One student, for example, emphasized the importance of respect but also felt that being casual, or even laughing about what was going on, was not disrespectful: "I think she [the donor] would have wanted us to enjoy it" (anonymous, interview, March 21, 2012).

A name is a linguistic framing, a title, a way of carving out an arena and an identity, of identifying figure from ground. Names give a donor a personality and a history in the face of imposed official anonymity, albeit a personality and history that is fictionalized and imagined. Fred and Joe can be imagined as having been "average Joes," while an Agnes or Herman become "fondly remembered old people" (Wright 2005). Even more joking and irreverent names such as "the Green Lantern" ascribe historical and cultural characteristics to the cadaver, doing exactly what official stances do not want: imputing humanity and life to a body that has been rationalized for medical purposes.

Imputing humanity or "living" traits to corpses exists in tradition more broadly. Folklorists and other scholars have documented narratives about practical jokes with corpses in wakes and other contexts (see Thursby 2006; Narváez 2003). Folklorist Ray Cashman (2006, 16) writes in a footnote that in Irish wakes of the past, "although clearly understood as dead in physical terms . . . the deceased used to be treated as alive in social terms." Historical photos provide evidence that medical students participated in versions of this tradition as well. One photo from the Boston Medical Library, for example, shows a medical student lying on the table about to be "dissected" by skeletons and corpses (figure 3.3); other similar historical "tomfoolery" medical

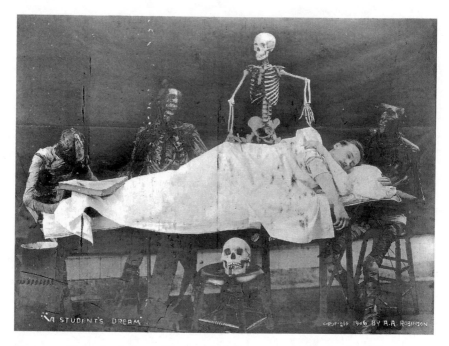

Figure 3.3. "A Student's Dream" by A. A. Robinson, 1910. Boston Medical Library. Photograph of student being "dissected" by corpses.

photos also exist. Giving the donor a name participates in this tradition of treating the dead as alive in social terms and is a linguistic rehumanization in the face of institutionalized dehumanization. Medical researchers Austin Williams and colleagues (2014, 175) similarly concluded that naming represented a deeper connection with the cadaver and an acknowledgment of the donor's humanity.

Another type of folklore that sometimes emerges in gross anatomy lab are apocryphal stories and legends, many of which are thought to be funny. Legends are stories or propositions about extraordinary events purported to be true and they describe highly unlikely but potentially real (as opposed to obviously fictional) events. Legends are not usually categorized as a form of humor, but as Tim Tangherlini (1996, 918) observes, the connection between legends and jokes is close, and he writes that prominent legend scholar Linda Dégh called the two forms "symbiotic." The majority of legends are fictional, but they straddle the boundary between fiction and nonfiction, being just plausible enough for tellers and listeners to ask themselves: could this extraordinary event be true?

Contemporary legends, which are one category of legend, address the anxieties and stressors of modern life.[8] Hafferty (1988, 1991) collected what he calls "cadaver stories" (contemporary legends) from students taking gross anatomy. One legend type he collected is a story in which the identity of the donor is revealed as a relative of a student doing the dissection.[9] In these legends, the donor usually is recognized on the first day of class, but in one variation, the donor is unrecognized until the end of the course, when the student takes the gauze off the face to ready the head for dissection. The student is shocked and horrified to discover that they have dissected a relative.

Some physicians I interviewed were familiar with legends about medical students and body donors. Dr. York, attended medical school in the late 1980s, told me the following legend about an alleged practical joke that circulated among medical students in Scotland at that time:

> **MY:** Actually, there was a story from my school that (I don't know if it's true or not), because there's always these—
> **LG:** It's folklore.
> **MY:** Urban legends—folklore [laughs], right—
> **MY:** Exactly. [I heard] that someone had chopped the tips of the fingers off of their cadaver . . . and gone to one of the buildings on campus that had an elevator. And as they were getting, while they waited until the doors were clos-ing, and then said, "Hold on, hold on," and then just as the doors were closing, they threw in the tips that they had—. . . And screamed, as the doors closed, into the elevator, with people in it. . . . And the story goes that—. . . This was complained about and he [the medical student] ended up getting expelled. . . . Which would be perfectly appropriate, but I don't know how true the story is.
> (Interview, September 6, 2018)

In this story, the medical student is a prankster who uses the donor's fingertips to play a practical joke.

Dr. Price recalled a similar legend. In this example, the student took the donor's bones out of the lab, but accidentally left them on public transportation.

> But there was a funny story, and I don't know if this ever happened for sure, but they would assign a bone box to each student (which was a human skeleton in like a wooden box) that you could take the bones out [of] and study the different kind of anatomical features of the bones. And somebody (apparently) took their bone box home and left it on the trolley—. . . And had forgotten it there, and that caused a bit of a raucous with the police. . . . So, after that, the bone boxes had to stay in the facility.
> (Interview, November 8, 2019)

A third physician I interviewed referred to a story kernel in which someone supposedly took home the head of a cadaver, although she did not elaborate on the nature of the tale.

All examples end with a shocking revelation, a common conclusion for contemporary legends. The shock evokes laughter. In the first narrative, the shock is that of the medical student who supposedly dissected a relative, while in the second and third stories, the shock is of a layperson who unexpectedly encounters human body parts in public left by trickster or careless medical students. Hafferty interprets cadaver legends as helping students emotionally socialize into their new roles as physicians through emotional modeling. According to this interpretation, the person who responds emotionally to the cadaver by becoming upset is held up in a negative light, while the detached, unemotional response (ideally held by medical students) is positive and to be emulated.

In my own view, these stories narratively violate official, institutionalized stances that advocate donor anonymity, respect, and proper care of bodies. Contemporary legends take an idea, value, or stance and exaggerate it or invert it to the point of near impossibility, making that idea more concrete and visible. The first example plays with the idea that donors are supposed to be anonymous. Body donations only work if the anatomist does not know the donor, and this example illustrates what might happen otherwise. The next examples illustrate what (allegedly) happens when body parts are removed from the semiprivate, medicalized, and rationalized environment of the lab and made public. The corpse is degraded, laughter erupts, and the core medical value of respect for the body donor is overturned. In addition, because the donor is the medical student's symbolic first patient, the sacrosanct nature of the doctor-patient relationship is violated. Such stories are carnivalesque because they treat dismemberment in a comic manner, they evoke laughter, and because they subvert official "aristocratic" core values and discourse. They also provide explicit moral warnings and so ultimately reaffirm and uphold those same institutionalized values. Dr. York commented: "And this is another aspect of the humor thing, it's a funny story in a way that practical jokes are funny, right? But you don't know how true it is, but has it served the purpose of warning to students, 'That got us expelled, don't do that'" (Interview, September 6, 2018).

These stories explore serious transgression, mediating in narrative what happens in the lab. As explained previously, Mary Douglas (1968) argues that jokes are symbolic representations of ruptures in social patterns. Students who engage in dissection violate taboos and engage in transgressive acts. Transgression in legend is merely made bigger and more dramatic: one dissects not just an anonymous donor but a beloved relative; one doesn't just remove a finger but takes fingers out of the lab and plays a practical joke with them. Telling these legends helps students "think" about the transgression of boundaries in a context in which actual boundaries are being violated. Such stories explore the questions, Where is the line? Which boundaries are acceptable to cross and which are not?

Other, more subtle kinds of humorous experiences also do this kind of boundary work. As dissection proceeds, what constitutes the body, what the body looks like, and what is appropriate to the body are redefined for students, and this reconceptualization emerges in many ways. For example, students found unexpected objects or unusual anatomical structures. Students identified tumors, black lungs of smokers, and other evidence of disease; these were expected. However, students also discovered man-made objects. They found breast, testicular, butt, and chest implants, which they did not expect and that sometimes elicited jokes or laughter. Students expected natural bodies and physiological processes, but they found evidence of human intervention. Donors still had pacemakers, which continued to function and sometimes went off, despite the fact that the recipient was no longer alive (Block 2004b). The donor may also have unexpected tattoos or other body modifications, or students discovered wires from medical devices embedded in the body as they dissected. Laughter arises around the incongruous and unexpected: we expect one thing and something else happens. These unexpected objects or surprising anatomical structures were a source of humor for medical students as what was unexpected about the body was revealed.

The most obvious cadaver folklore that illustrated redefinitions of the human body were stories, analogies, and allusions associating cadavers with food. These examples are the most carnivalesque folklore that emerge in gross anatomy because they treat the anatomized, dismembered body in a culinary manner; Bakhtin writes specifically that "the anatomic and culinary treatment [found in carnival imagery] is based on the grotesque image of the dissected body" ([1968] 1984, 194). Hafferty collected several legend examples. In one variant, the cadaver becomes a receptacle: "Candy, potato chips, or other types of food are hidden in body cavities, ready to be hauled out and consumed in front of unsuspecting viewers." In another, "students transform an eviscerated abdomen into a gigantic lunchtime salad bowl" by lining it with tinfoil and putting vegetables in it (1988, 348; see also Hafferty 1991). In some legends students actually ate the cadaver, but more often they simply associated the cadaver with food in order to prank another student, who fainted in response and whom, according to Hafferty, was worthy of ridicule as they had not demonstrated the proper professional demeanor of detachment.

I did not find such legends in my research (I did not ask for them specifically), but there definitely was an association between cadavers and food both
in oral interviews and the literature. Humans are a form of animal protein as
Richard Selzer, a well-known physician and writer, made explicit in his famous
1975 essay "The Corpse":

> Commonplace food!
> Turned Meat! Spangled leftovers!
> Blue-plate special served too late!

Students struggled to make sense of what they dissected, and they sometimes
did so by translating unfamiliar structures into familiar images of food. One
medical student explained, "I think we're all kind of trying to disassociate from
the whole situation, so I think you know, a lot of people would see the muscle and
be like, 'Wow, that looks a lot like meat,' or you know—things that are really not
appropriate when you repeat them, but kind of gets you through . . . through the
situation" (anonymous, interview, March 22, 2012). When NPR's Melissa Block
asked one medical student to describe a nerve he had just dissected, the student,
surprised at how big the nerve actually was, responded, "It kind of looks like a
piece of pasta in some ways. I think that's kind of uh, you know, like a piece of
spaghetti—maybe a little bit bigger? Maybe a little bit flatter?" (Block 2004a).
Students melted the donor's fat in order to complete a particular step, which was
then difficult not to imagine as melted butter, or grease. The fact that humans can
be eaten became visible and concrete as anatomical structures were dissected.

One result of this revelation was that some medical students (at least initially) experienced difficulties eating certain foods. A medical student I interviewed stated, "It seemed like all the analogies we made [were] like, 'Oh, that
looks like melted butter; that looks like oatmeal.' And it was always food. And
I'm like, 'Oh, there's another thing I can't eat anymore'" (anonymous, interview,
March 22, 2012). One student commented in *The First Patient* (2018), "You sort
of realize this chicken that I'm eating, it has a lot of the same parts as a person.
It sort of made me want to be a vegetarian." Others had the opposite reaction:
one physician I interviewed recalled that her lab group, in a somewhat oppo-
sitionally defiant move, purposefully went out for steaks after lab. The theme
that dissection interfered with one's ability to eat also showed up in medical
blogs. The following excerpt was written by a medical student whose donor was
riddled with cancerous tumors:

> We were supposed perform a hysterectomy, but our group had trouble even
> finding the uterus. At first, we attempted to remove the tumor, which we
> later found out had engulfed the left ovary and was about the size of a Nerf

football. After removing it, our group then split up into "let's see what is
inside a tumor" and "let's find the rest of the female pelvic anatomy." I, for
one, was completely grossed out by just removing the tumor (i.e. it will be
a long time before I eat tuna fish again), and so I opted for the latter group,
all the while focusing my eyes away from the tumor dissection and the
discovery of the "chocolate cyst" within it. It is one thing for anatomy to end
my love of tuna fish . . . but I could not bear to let it prevent me from eating
chocolate. (Gold 2011)

There also was anxiety about ingesting or inhaling cadaver material. This
fear of accidental ingestion was not entirely conjectural. At certain points during dissection, for example, students use the bone saw, which sends small bone
chips and bone dust into the air. Students must keep their mouths closed while
using the bone saw to avoid getting cadaver material in their mouths or breathing the dust into the lungs. My spouse told me a story about one of his lab
partners who talked continuously throughout their lab. When it was time to
use the bone saw, he warned everyone at the table to keep their mouths closed.
The lab partner continued to talk despite the warning. My partner turned the
bone saw on, threw up the expected chips and dust, and the lab partner got
cadaver material in his mouth, generating hilarity and ridicule from his peers.

Folkloric connections between cadavers and food closely parallel themes of
anatomization and dismemberment in relation to feasting prevalent in ancient
carnivalesque images. The grotesque body is imagined as a collective, cosmic
body that is dismembered and eaten in all kinds of popular-festive forms. A
focus on the open, swallowing mouth that feasts on another, dismembered
body, alongside a strong focus on the belly and the digestive system bring into
sharp relief the material bodily processes of life and death (Bakhtin [1968]
1984, 317). Culinary images commonly accompanied descriptions of battle
scenes in Rabelais's works. Battlefields were described as kitchens or linked
to images of banquets, and descriptions of bodies torn asunder by war were
described in food-related terms. Bakhtin ([1968] 1984, 193–94) alludes to a
description by Rabelais of a battle in which Friar John—described as a "systemic
'anatomizer'"—kills 13,622 men. The rent bodies are treated in a "culinary fash-
ion" as images of blood are tuned into wine, since the battle is to save the mon-
astery's new crop of grapes (209). Bakhtin writes, "It is a bodily sowing, or more
correctly speaking a bodily harvest. . . . There is a combination of the battlefield
with the kitchen or butcher shop" (207). Graphic descriptions of beatings are
similar, such as the beatings of the catchpoles, in which eyes and ears and bones
are turned to pulp: "We see once more the anatomizing dismemberment and
the culinary and medical terms which accompany it" (202).

Conceptualizing human cadavers as food also brings up deeply rooted fears of contamination and defilement (Douglas [1966] 2003). Mary Douglas observes that both the body and food constitute the cultural order. The body constitutes a bounded system that stands for the social order, while the margins and orifices of the body, like the mouth, are points of entry that need protection. Similarly, what constitutes food also reflects the social order. Douglas explains in her well-known analysis of the abominations of Leviticus that items that are forbidden to eat are anomalous, standing outside the normal order of classification. Like dirt, they are matter out of place (36). Such items are polluting and to consume them is to invite danger and defilement. As the body constitutes the social order so should what is eaten also reflect social and cultural coherency.

Food scholars have drawn on Douglas's work to unpack connections between eating and the maintenance of boundaries between self and not-self. Uneaten food may be coded as "other" or "dead," but a transformation occurs once food is eaten: food then becomes "self" and "life-giving" as the not-self becomes self (Roth 2017). The maintenance of boundaries between self and other also is why disgust can be a response to food (Bronner 1981): food may be perceived as being either "too alien" from the self (e.g., bugs in some cultures) or too close, such as pets or people (Korsmeyer 2002, 219). Pollution or contamination occurs if such food is eaten because the social order has been violated. A body donor that is perceived as both "human" and "food" as happens in gross anatomy folklore profoundly upsets regular orders of classification. A cadaver is "too close" to be food: a person who eats a cadaver is contaminated, and presumably anyone who thinks of a cadaver as food-like risks contamination.

If both the human body and food represent the social order and the act of eating entails the transformation of the not-self to self through ingestion and absorption, then to imagine a human body as food is to imagine violating the social order and standing completely outside of it. Food scholar LuAnne Roth suggested in a personal communication that it is as if the students are placed in the position of a monster, such as a zombie, a creature known to dine on human flesh and who often exist because of contamination. A monster defies natural categories and orders of classification, and they may be symbols of defilement. Monsters also often have unusual or unnatural powers because of their marginality. Such imaginings make concrete what Young (1997) calls unstable binaries: self and other; human and not-human; student and lab specimen; life and death. In this imagery, the students become completely anomalous (outside of classification) and risk defilement, echoing the students' actual social situation as they move through anatomy class and learn to engage routinely in transgressive but medically sanctioned acts.

Humor plays an important role by keeping such ideas from becoming obscenity. Douglas (1968) perceived close similarities between jokes and pollution. As noted in the introduction, she characterized jokes as "anti-rites" because they disorganize society and destroy hierarchy and order in a manner similar to pollution. But the humorous utterance required by the rupture in social context only makes a little disturbance as it mirrors the ruptured social situation. It remains restricted by social consensus. Obscenity, in contrast, totally opposes social structure, which is why it is offensive. Allusions to cadavers as food then, reflect the existing situation as transgressive or paradoxical, but help control it. In the gross lab, seemingly juvenile cadaver stories and visual food analogies become meditations on cultural categories of the world and the order of things.

Sexual jokes, comments, and asides also arise during gross anatomy class. Themes of sex and its interrelationship to death are ancient. The Oedipal legend cycle, in which Oedipus unknowingly murders his father Laius and marries his mother Jocosta, is the most famous example. Genesis 19 also connects sex and death through the obliteration of Sodom and Gomorrah. It is obvious but bears repeating that cadavers are naked. Students confront death as a naked body, and according to Hafferty (1988, 351), "many are disturbed by the sight (or anticipated sight) of so much nakedness, not to mention the sight of so many penises, vaginas, breasts, and nipples permanently shorn of their sensuality by death." There are, for example, apocryphal stories about medical students who cut off the penis of their cadaver and insert it into the vagina of a nearby lab cadaver; about students who supposedly link two whole cadavers in a sexual embrace; or students who fit a condom to a male cadaver's penis (Hafferty 1988, 347). A folklore colleague of mine related a legend he heard from his best friend whose brother was in medical school at Washington University in St. Louis sometime between 1963 and 1968 (note the "close-but-distant" authenticating source that indicates the tale is a contemporary legend). The story states that one day the brother and his lab partners uncovered their cadaver to find a severed penis in the vagina. (It was unclear from the story whether the students discovered this or whether they were the perpetrators of the joke.) They showed the cadaver to their female instructor (as my colleague commented, gender is a critical element of the story), who then quipped, "Well, I see one of you left in a hurry last night" (for a published variation of this story, see Thorson 1993). Such overt "cadaver antics" largely are apocryphal, although one doctor told me that in her gross anatomy class she cut off her donor's penis as part of the dissection and then stuck it in the kidney as a joke (anonymous, personal communication, October 3, 2019).

The dissection of the cadaver's genitalia can be one of the most uncomfortable parts of dissection for students, what Reifler (1996, 190) calls the "brutalization of their [the students'] cultural norms." Students must cut off the penis if their donor is male or completely dissect the vulva if the donor is female. The dissection of the penis was particularly difficult for male students (Segal 1988, 22) and the entire pelvic unit can lead to off-color comments. One student explained:

> **M1:** Doing the pelvis unit—[there were] definitely a lot of sexual jokes in the anatomy lab.
> **LG:** Uh-huh? Can you remember any of them, specifically?
> **M1:** There was—I mean, like there were a lot of those—have you heard of "That's what she said" jokes?
> **LG:** I vaguely remember these, but can you remind me?
> **M1:** Yeah, it's pretty much like you could turn anything into a sexual innuendo. . . . If you say like, "This is hard." Like, *That's what she said.*
> (Anonymous, interview, March 21, 2012)

When I asked the student for more examples, they responded: "Like we were dissecting the female's (we had a female cadaver), so we were trying to dissect her genitalia. And one of my lab mates said, 'I'll get between her legs.' 'Get between her legs,'... —it was like if you said this in real life, like someone would just like jump" (anonymous, interview, March 21, 2012).

There also are published examples that address humor, death, and sex in gross anatomy lab. At Northwestern University Medical School, students are encouraged to write essay responses to gross anatomy, participating in the field of narrative medicine founded by Rita Charon designed to help medical students deal with their emotions and counter detachment through writing. In one assignment, students wrote about dissection from their cadavers' point of view. Reifler (1996, 192) writes that in some student stories the cadavers maintained their composure and sense of humor throughout dissection, which they (the cadavers) found to be unpleasant: "Regarding dissection of his genitals by one of the female medical students [the cadaver states]: 'I suppose I shouldn't be surprised by anything at this point. You're all animals. Let's get on with it.'"

Other examples do not necessarily have to do with the genitals per se but rather with intimate bodily parts and processes that are taboo in ordinary conversation. One medical student I interviewed told the following story:

> They [medical students] are dealing with something that could potentially be rather uncomfortable for a lot of people. So I think that sort of situation

where you can express yourself and you're dealing with an uncomfortable situation makes it a really great spot to use humor to kind of cope what's going on. For instance, I remember with my anatomy group we had four girls and one guy and when we got down to the abdomen, the proctor told us that we would have to put a tampon in the anus to prevent leakage of some really malodorous fluid. So all the girls were all like, well, we all know how to do this I think you should—the guy—should do it. So we told the guy to do it. And then we he looked at the anus and there were external hemorrhoids. And he's like, "This does not look like any butt that I've ever seen. I don't know how to do this." [Laughter.] (Anonymous, interview, April 10, 2012)

The death-related folklore that emerges in gross anatomy is a carnivalesque response to the complex situation in which medical students find themselves. Dissection and gross anatomy exist within a modern cultural context that denies death and in which people rarely see dead bodies. As the cadaver is dissected, students come to know and understand the human body on the most intimate of levels but, in doing so, the students transgress serious social and cultural norms that they will continue to break in various ways over the course of their career. These transgressions place them in an ambivalent position and at risk of defilement. Further, the gross lab seeks to construct a professional medical identity by reorienting students' responses to death and the patient's body from lay responses to rationalized and technocratic orientations. A carnivalesque response resists this ongoing instrumentalization and rationalization while directly acknowledging the taboos and boundaries that are consistently crossed.

The connections I make here between anatomy and carnival exist historically: dissection and the dissected body are carnivalesque. Renate Lachmann (1988–89, 147) notes that "the medicine of the Renaissance also displays a new interest in the body, as, for example, in the dissection of corpses and the meticulous description of pathologies. This has its carnivalesque pendant in the gay dismemberment of bodies, in the ridiculing of death, and in the obscene exposure of the body." Not only was anatomization an aspect of Rabelais's writings, as noted previously, but also public dissections in Bologna literally were associated with Carnival during the Renaissance (Ferrari 1987, 66). In the 1500s, public dissections came to be scheduled in January, during Carnival, which was when students took holidays. Later in the century, it was decreed that anatomy was to be done during the Christmas and Carnival periods to help preserve the bodies, and so for a period there was an overt association between dissection and festivity. Historian Giovanna Ferrari points out that public dissections were a spectacle, almost like a theatrical production. People sometimes came in masks and occasionally grew unruly. And, returning to relations between food and anatomization, Ferrari writes that the fat from publicly dissected corpses was sometimes used in pharmaceuticals. While the situation and context in modern anatomy labs obviously is quite different, the profound ambivalence of the carnivalesque, grounded in the materiality of death, reemerges in modern contexts as a useful and relevant orientation for students as they navigate a difficult class.

Beyond Anatomy: Other Death-Related Folklore

A physician's relationship with death begins, but does not end, in the gross anatomy lab. Peter Finkelstein and Lawrence Mathers (1990, 220) write, "The dissection of the body is usually the first in a long series of encounters with death" in a physician's lifetime. Gross anatomy socializes medical students into interacting intimately with death and the body in a routine manner, but the specter of death haunts physicians throughout their career.

Anthropologist Anne Burson-Tolpin (1989, 287) observes that doctors sometimes shift into what she calls "alternating register play" when speaking about death, meaning that physicians may speak in a style that is more playful than their regular, serious, and official speech styles. One of the most common ways in which this playful register is deployed is through the use of slang, which may occur in hospital contexts. Slang is difficult to define but sometimes is characterized as "informal" speech (Peterson 1998; Coombs et al. 1993). Slang consists of terms that are purposefully low register, meaning that they stand in opposition to official, formal, or more dignified forms of speaking by being of a distinctly lesser status. This is in part because slang historically was associated with the speech of the lower (presumably disreputable) classes and it is common among tight-knit groups, including prisons, gangs, and the military. Today it is recognized that people of all social classes may use slang, but slang itself continues to be contrasted with official, polite speech and associated with notions of disrepute. As an informal, low-register manner of speaking then, slang is a useful way to accomplish carnivalesque subversions of official stances toward death.

Certainly not all physicians use slang: many doctors are ambivalent about its use and so the use of slang is conflicted (Parsons et al. 2001). There are, however, slang terms for death that are widely known among medical personnel and are easily available through published surveys, websites, blogs, books, and collectanea (Coombs et al. 1993; Fox et al. 2003; Becker 1993; Gordon 1983). Examples include the following:

- Coded
- Turned in his lunch basket
- Out at the plate
- Bought the farm/bought it
- Joined the air force
- Go down the tubes

Slang terms for death are not limited to the United States. In one survey of doctors in Great Britain, for example, physician Adam Fox and colleagues (2003) elicited the following:

- DOA: dead on arrival
- FUBAR: fucked up beyond all repair
- GPO: good for parts only
- Pathology outpatients: refers to mortuary
- Rose cottage: refers to mortuary
- T.F. BUNDY: totally fucked but unfortunately not dead yet
- Circling the drain
- Coffin dodger: old person

And a website that documented slang terms in both the US and Great Britain (Messybeast, n.d.) listed the following:

- Angel lust: male corpse with an erection
- ART: approaching room temperature
- AST: assuming seasonal temperature
- Cancel Christmas
- Cold tea syndrome: refers to the several cups of tea beside a dead patient
- Death star—that ward in every hospital where patients die
- DRT: dead right there (at scene of accident)
- DRTTT: dead right there and there and there and there: that is, scattered at multiple parts of the accident
- DWPA: death with paramedic assistance

- ECU: eternal care unit
- FDSTW: found dead, stayed that way
- GTMJACB: gone to meet Jesus, ain't coming back
- ITBNTL: in the box, nail the lid
- Code purple: when paramedics are called out to a dead body

Many additional terms are available online for the curious reader.

These terms often imitate medical jargon or medical acronyms. The phrase "gone to the ECU (eternal care unit)," for example, mimics the acronym ICU, which stands for the intensive care unit. This mimicry is the basis of the subversiveness. A "code purple," which means someone has died, imitates hospital codes. Codes are emergency declarations, sometimes made over the hospital speaker system (or to pagers or apps on phones) that often are associated with a color. A code red, for example, refers to a fire; a code blue means the heart or breathing has stopped, and a code orange is a hazardous spill. There is no standardized code for purple but a "code purple" presumably refers to the color of someone who has died. The code is humorous because, unlike real codes, no immediate emergency action is necessary. (Such a code would never go over a speaker or other formal system but only emerge in spoken conversation.)

Other types of slang parody formal diagnosis. These phrases are funny both because of their imitative nature and because they describe the condition of death, so the medical diagnosis is unnecessary. The phrase "cold tea syndrome" refers to someone who has died and therefore has one or more cups of cold tea at their bedside that they did not drink. To say that someone is a "pathology outpatient" is absurd: pathology has no patient contact because pathologists work with tissue samples and bodies. A pathology outpatient by definition is someone who is dead.

Slang and slang-like terms replace an official, formal, or more dignified term with a term that is "lower." This replacement presumes knowledge of the official term and expands meaning for both the higher and the lower term by bringing them into relation with each other. Slang functions as metaphor, which create meaning by bringing disparate elements together. Each element takes on the other's characteristics, expanding the ranges of significance. To refer to a particular hospital ward as the "death star," for example, brings that ward into alignment with the Death Star from the *Star Wars* films. The Death Star was a mobile space station and a powerful weapon of the Galactic Empire designed to destroy planets. To refer to a hospital ward as the Death Star is to impute the qualities of the *Star Wars* Death Star to a particular hospital section and implies that the patients sent there have, like the Rebels, little hope of return or escape. It does not target patients but, rather, the ward's expertise or, more pointedly, alleged lack thereof.

There are visual jokes about death, although these are less common. One well-known example is the O and Q sign (figure 3.4), first put into print in *The House of God*, but which presumably existed prior to that publication. These signs refer to the patient's mouth and also parody diagnosis. In the visual, if a patient's mouth is open in the shape of a round O for a long period of time, the prognosis is dire. If a patient leaves their mouth open with the tip of the tongue hanging out (hence, a Q shape, the tail of the Q being the tongue), the patient is close to death. As Fats says in *The House of God*, "The O SIGN is reversible, but once they get to the Q SIGN, they never come back" (Shem [1978] 2003, 230).

The O and Q sign can become even more inappropriate, as in the "dotted Q." The dotted Q is a classic Q sign with a fly on the end of the tongue (thus dotting the tail of the Q), indicating that the patient died quite some time ago. There also is the "QT" sign, which means that the tongue is out, and the tablet remains on the end of it (Fox et al. 2003, 187). One blogger with the username 911doc explained the O and Q diagnosis in an online discussion thread (911doc 2008), which was followed by extended commentary from other physicians about whether or not it was ethical to talk about patients in this way. One poster sunnily responded on June 6, 2008: "Cheer up 911 [the original blogger]. The 'O' sign isn't limited to the near dead; *I occasionally display this sign myself.* Then there's the 'dotted O' sign, when there's an endotracheal tube in the middle of the O—again, not always terminal" (italics mine).[10]

Joking about death emerges in private with other physicians in socially situated contexts of difficult work, and such conversations are difficult to document. When I asked for examples in interviews, physicians naturally were reluctant to talk about them. One physician, however, shared an example. As a psychiatrist, they deal with issues of mental health, including suicide ideation. Psychiatrists do everything they can to keep their patients from committing suicide, but patient suicide does occur and is a real threat. Alternatively, sometimes patients attempt suicide and fail. This particular physician had a teenage patient who allegedly tried to commit suicide by standing under the shower, looking up, and opening their mouth, thinking they would drown. Given this spectacularly unsuccessful attempt, it is not surprising that the patient's physicians found it amusing. When the patient was discussed during rounds, the doctor noted that the failed attempt led to comments about turkeys looking up, since turkeys supposedly do this and can drown when it rains. They followed this story with the comment, "Who says things like that?!? Horrible people" (personal communication, January 14, 2020).

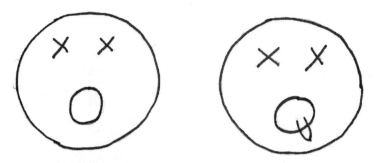

Figure 3.4. O and Q sign. Illustration by author in imitation of Samuel Shem.

Are doctors horrible people because some of them occasionally engage in death-related folklore? The answer is no. Physicians are quite human though, despite society's attempts to place them on pedestals as gods and heroes. Irreverent and playful attitudes toward death also exist outside of medicine, both today and in the past (see Narváez 2003). One early example of "graveyard humor" can be found in Shakespeare's *Hamlet,* in which the gravediggers are clowns who exchange witticisms, riddles, and puns; they also sing and drink as they dig (act V, scene 1). Premodern Irish wakes are a classic example, and even today, it is common for storytelling and laughter to occur among participants downstairs, alongside the more serious and sober conversations that occur in the room with the actual body (Cashman 2006). Folklorist Jacqueline Thursby (2006) catalogs what she calls "frivolities around death" in the US, which includes not only humor at Irish American wakes but also funny stories from funeral directors, legend trips to cemeteries, *calaveras* and laughing skeletons of Day of the Dead celebrations, and humorous epitaphs. Humor about death also emerges in popular culture. Folklorist Trevor Blank (2013) examines jokes about celebrity and mass mediated disasters as they play out on the internet, while folklorist Montana Miller (2012) researches how students play with the idea of death in her examination of staged high school drunk driving accidents that purport to educate students. Connections between playfulness and death then, are traditional, despite (or because of) the fact that death is a taboo topic.

Physicians' daily work is suffused with issues of death. Physicians work with the sick and dying in difficult situations that can cause them to suffer. Their professional duty directs them to save people from sickness and death, while at the same time the general cultural context forbids them from speaking about death and frames death as a failure, a loss, and a tragedy that is always to be taken seriously. Physicians also are supposed to respond to death and the body in technocratic and rationalized ways, creating tensions between the difficult reality of those experiences, the professional stance they are supposed to inhabit, and the larger cultural milieu. Slang and related forms of playful speech offer a way out of, and alternative to, the formal, official or monologic speech in which physicians must engage, expanding the ranges of meaning for death by reframing it as something else. C. Peterson (1998) argues that the extensive existence of slang terms among physicians in Brazil means that there is an ethos expressed by medical slang that is not available in other registers, although exactly what that ethos signifies is unclear, since slang is connotative rather than denotative. Alternatively, Coombs and colleagues (1993, 995) suggest that humorous slang about death functions to soften tragedy and can "veil the harshness of medical life," while at the same time being an exercise in wit. Douglas (1968, 374) suggested that a joke itself "mimics a kind of death." My own view is that death-related folklore and humorous shop-talk participate in a carnivalesque orientation that works directly against occupational directives of rationalism and professionalism, as well as the ethos of stoicism, seriousness, silence, and heroism that permeate medical culture, all of which seek to mute or downplay the fact that death is a part of life.

Notes

1. *Gomerpedia*, s.v., "Death," last edited August 8, 2017, http://gomerpedia .org/index.php?title=Death&action=history.

2. Interestingly, some of these modern movements echo an older way of thinking about death that Ariès described; in this older model, a dying person knew the hour of their death or actively died at a specific time because the person, not the physician, was the active agent and in control.

3. Anatomists in Arabia, the most famous of which was Avicenna, significantly advanced medical knowledge during this period.

4. The University of Padua built an anatomy theater in 1595.

5. The practice of grave robbing was so prevalent that people with financial means built graves with iron bars or springs on the coffin lid designed to deter thieves. See dethorne 2015.

6. The Burke case was so famous and public outcry so strong that broadside ballads were composed about the event.

7. The treatment of body donations by third parties in the US, however, apparently remains somewhat unregulated and problematic. See Grow and Shiffman 2017.

8. The Utah State University Fife Folklore Archives categorizes legends as follows: (1) character legends, or legends about famous historical figures; (2) supernatural nonreligious legends; (3) religious legends; (4) etiological legends, which are origin stories; (5) legends about the human condition, such as legends about migration and slavery; and (6) contemporary legends. Contemporary legends are legends that circulate about the dangers of modern life and provide warnings or moral admonitions.

9. Hafferty (1991, 56–58) identified five types of contemporary legends about cadavers in his research, although he does not identify them as contemporary legends but rather as stories. They are: (1) stories in which students carry cadavers or cadaver parts outside to the lab for shock purposes; (2) stories about the manipulation of sexual organs; (3) stories in which the cadaver appears to be alive; (4) stories in which the cadaver is identified as a relative or friend; and (5) stories of cadavers as food.

10. Some minor editing for spelling and punctuation added for clarity.

4

Bodies of Humor

The Medicalized and the Grotesque

The interesting thing about medicine and the human body is that nothing in the human body really becomes . . . off-limits.

—Anonymous, interview, March 21, 2012

When physicians get together, they talk about work, and they tell stories of cases that they came across personally or heard about from peers. These stories often focus on strange or unusual things about the human body. Many of these stories are funny, while others stretch the boundaries of the imagination by focusing on the bizarre or unusual. They can also be a combination of both.

My father-in-law Dr. William Walsh was an orthopedic surgeon in New York and had several such stories in his repertoire. The following narrative he told is apocryphal, closer to a legend than a personal experience narrative, but it illustrates a kind of story that doctors tell about funny, weird, or strange bodily events. This story allegedly happened at Lenox Hill Hospital in New York City and was told to him while he was a medical student in the mid-1960s.

> When I was a medical student, I used to work nights, part-time at Lenox Hill Hospital, on Park Avenue. But I would hang out with the interns and residents there, so they kind of—I'd find out from them what was going on. And I was treated like I was part of the housestaff, even though I was still a student.
>
> But at any rate, one of the stories I remember from that place is that there was a fellow who was walking Park Avenue, and there was somebody having a cocktail party several stories up, in the luxury apartment house there. And probably one of the guests at the cocktail party dropped a champagne glass

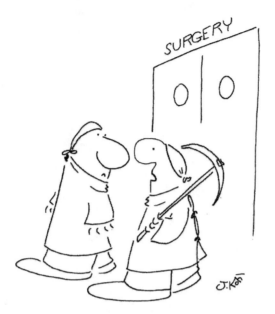

"Ever see gall stones like that before?"

Figure 4.1. Cartoon commenting on surgical finding of unusual size.

out the window. And this fellow walking along the sidewalk suddenly felt what he described as a sudden onset of a severe, splitting headache.

And he walked into the emergency room at Lenox Hill Hospital, which was on Park Avenue, saying, "I've got this severe headache; it just came on very suddenly, and it feels like it's just splitting my head."

And the intern looks at him, and he's got this champagne glass sticking out of the top of his head. I guess the base had shattered—. . . And the stem was stuck right in the top of his skull. (Interview, February 15, 2015)

Like all good legends, this narrative tests the boundaries of believability by tacking back and forth between truth and fiction. It is cloaked in a rhetoric of truth (Oring 2008), which exists in narrative markers like "When I was a medical student" and direct dialogue that present an "I was there, I know people who saw it" perspective that enhances believability. The content is almost-but-not-quite-unbelievable, which makes it an appealing story.

Such extraordinary stories overlap with more realistic ones, making boundaries between legend and personal experience fuzzy. Common examples include personal experience narratives about complex patients whose bodies did not follow presumed pathology.[1] Surgeons might tell stories of operations where a patient's anatomy wasn't in the presumed place, complicating the surgery, as several surgeons explained to me in interviews. ER doctors tell stories of unbelievable physical trauma similar to ones told by first responders (Tangherlini 1998). Physicians-in-training tell of doing the unimaginable. When my partner was a second-year internal medicine resident in the ICU at the University of Utah, for example, an eighteen-year-old patient came in who had been shot in the chest. The bullet had pierced the aorta and stunned the heart. There was no reliable heartbeat: shock and chest compressions were not working. The surgery residents were doing other surgeries. The attending cardiothoracic surgeon also was not immediately available. Instead, he directed my spouse over the phone how to cut open the patient's chest and massage the heart with his hand in order to keep the patient alive until he arrived. He did, having never seen the procedure before. The patient survived; my partner was razzed for having cut through the man's nipple.

The body unites many physician-based narratives of work—what has been done to it through accident, disease, neglect, or on purpose—and what happened to that body once it entered the hospital. This talk includes not only narratives, but also jokes, quips, humorous asides, and other folklore forms. It can be coarse and includes themes of excretion, bodily fluids, physical size, abnormalities, and other topics taboo in modern, everyday conversation.

In this chapter, I argue that ancient notions of the grotesque body underlie this talk. The term *grotesque* here does not mean "gross" or "disgusting" or "ugly" in the modern sense of the term but rather refers to a metaphorical and aesthetic system of ideas. The grotesque body is innately associated with carnival and the carnivalesque. It is relentlessly material, based largely in the life- and death-related processes of the lower torso such as copulation, birth, digestion, and defecation. It is also uncontained, exaggerated, and generative. The grotesque body is ambivalent, transgressive, and generates laughter, and it is the basis on which alternative meanings are posited.

The grotesque body is difficult for contemporary audiences to grasp because it is counterintuitive to modern ideas. Modern ideas about the body are similar to what Bakhtin calls the "classical" body: in this framework, the body is individual rather than collective, closed as opposed to open, and a completed object rather than an unfinished entity. In contrast, the grotesque body is collective (even cosmic) rather than individual, and a primary characteristic is that it transgresses its own boundaries and fuses with other objects. For example, the grotesque body is associated with the mouth and acts of eating and swallowing, which mingle the body with the outer world. Another way in which the grotesque body transcends its own limits is through acts such as spitting, urinating, defecating, and vomiting—though not, apparently, through menstruating. Bakhtin's ([1968] 1984, 317) description is worth quoting at length:

> The grotesque body, as we have often stressed, is a body in the act of becoming. It is never finished, never completed; it is continually built, created, and builds and creates another body. Moreover, the body swallows the world and is itself swallowed by the world. . . . This is why the essential role belongs to those parts of the grotesque body in which it outgrows its own self, transgressing its own body, in which it conceives a new second body: the bowels and the phallus. . . . Next to the bowels and the genital organs is the mouth, through which enters the world to be swallowed up. And next is the anus. All these convexities and orifices have a common characteristic; it is within them that the confines between bodies and between the body and the world are overcome: there is an interchange and an interorientation. This is why the main events in the life of the grotesque body, the acts of the bodily drama, take place in this sphere. Eating, drinking, defecation and other elimination . . . as well as copulation, pregnancy, dismemberment, swallowing up by another body—all these acts are performed on the confines of the body and the outer world, or on the confines of the old and new body. In all these events the beginning and end of life are closely linked and interwoven.

While aspects of the grotesque body may appear "gross" in the modern sense of the world (that is, yucky), in tradition the grotesque body is viewed ambivalently as it synthesizes what Bakhtin calls the "positive and negative poles" (that is, positive and negative aspects of existence, such as life and death). The grotesque body appears "gross" to modern sensibilities because many aspects, such as its association with filth, oaths, curses, abuse, and the like, have lost their ancient affiliations with growth and renewal and have retained more narrow, solely negative meanings.

The grotesque body contrasts with the normative medicalized body, which is closely linked to issues of power. Michel Foucault foregrounds ideas about power and the body in works such as *The Birth of the Clinic* (1973) and *Discipline and Punish* (1977). Foucault links the rise of a new form of power at the end of the eighteenth century, which he calls "disciplinary power," to the new ways in which bodies were regulated in a variety of emerging institutions, including teaching hospitals. He contrasts disciplinary power to the older form of sovereign power, which resided in the body of the king or head of state and relied on public forms of terror. Both kinds of power are used to control. But in the newer, emerging institutions that used disciplinary power, bodies were arranged spatially, their activities organized, and elementary parts coordinated (McHoul and Grace 1997, 68–69): "The human body was entering a machinery of power that explores it, breaks it down, and rearranges it" (Foucault quoted in McHoul and Grace 1997, 68).

Teaching hospitals played an important role in the rise of disciplinary power as medicine came to govern aspects of biological life such as birth, death, sexual relations, sickness, and disease. Medicine in Europe was reorganized after the French Revolution, and teaching hospitals were established that were supposed to embody the revolution's liberating themes. These new hospitals led to the "birth of the clinic" meaning the birth of the clinical approach, which entailed new forms of observation, description, and language about the body. Thomas Osborne (1994, 34) observes that "the apotheosis of the clinic lies, then, with a mode of patient, laborious, qualitative description that is simultaneously a 'way of saying' and a 'way of seeing'; a form of discourse and a particular kind of gaze." The clinical approach was based on a privileging of perception, the surface of things, and the individual patient, including an orientation "to the individual case" and "a presentation of symptoms and . . . the patient's history" (Osborne 1994, 32). The clinical approach, along with the increased use of dissection, produced new knowledges about and definitions of the body.[2] The medical encounter today is understood as an event in which power is strategically deployed through techniques such as the interview, the case presentation, and the stethoscope, and scholars generally consider the body as not merely a given, taken-for-granted, biological entity but one that is produced in certain ways through such encounters. The body therefore is constituted by a variety of discourses and practices and is a site of struggle over the production of meaning (see Lupton 2003).[3]

Control over the body in medicine extends beyond patients to the bodies of physicians, a fact less often recognized. Good physicians are expected to control themselves, including their emotions. Emotional responses to the bodies of others are deemed "unprofessional," and certainly no one wants an emergency room physician to respond hysterically when confronted with trauma. Panic, disgust, fear, dread, and sadness are appropriate for laypeople confronted with disease and sickness, but emotions are not professionally appropriate for medical staff. Control of both the patient and physician body, accomplished through rationalist, reductionist models, objectification, and emotional containment, is a fundamental aspect of modern scientific medicine (see chap. 3).

The grotesque body offers an alternative to the controlled, medicalized body. Like the medicalized body, the grotesque body stands in relation to power but as a form of resistance, challenging disciplinary power. It does so through its own, undisciplined, transgressive body, the use of degradation, and rough speech. The grotesque body is chaotic and ambivalent, and it can produce laughter because it interrupts the primary directive of physician work, which is to control the body to produce good health.

Doctors and other medical personnel of course do not have an overt, conscious conception of the grotesque body in their everyday thinking. They are concerned with the practical management of patient bodies and physiology on a daily level. Physicians control patient bodies through surgery, medications, prescriptions for physical therapy, and mental exercises, but patient bodies can be unruly and do surprising, unexpected, or uncontrollable things. Cancer cells may grow despite radiation and treatment; weight returns to unhealthy levels despite regimes of diet and exercise; blood sugar and cholesterol levels rise despite medication.

Medical talk latently acknowledges the existence of an uncontrolled, grotesque body. Such talk is disciplining, meaning that it serves at the symbolic level to bring patient bodies back into line with idealized medical norms by noting how and where corporeal transgressions lie. Talk that indexes the grotesque body ultimately reinforces official hierarchies and patriarchal norms by positing the opposite. As Neil Ravenscroft and Paul Gilchrist (2009, 36) argue, "Carnivalesque inversions . . . are deployed to maintain and reinforce social order and, thus, the discipline of bodies and behaviors." The grotesque body is, however, a means through which an undisciplined, transgressive patient body is imagined and understood, and many ancient aspects of the grotesque body, such as associations with filth and abuse, emerge in medical talk. Medical folklore about the body therefore mediates between the biomedical ideal of a tightly controlled patient body and the realities of undisciplined, chaotic bodies that do not "mind" (Gabbert and Salud 2009).

It is important to note that the grotesque body has nothing to do with individuals. Katharine Young (1997) demonstrates how physician-patient interactions co-construct the body as an object for medical purposes; individual subjectivity and personhood are elided or reconstructed elsewhere. The body-oriented talk in which physicians engage is not about patients as individual human beings but about the biological situation. This separation of the body as an object from the individual has a long tradition in medicine.[4] Erika Brady (2001) points out that modern biomedical approaches are rooted in the history of Western intellectual thought, grounded in a Cartesian mind/body split and a reliance on empirical methods. A collective, grotesque body is an ambivalent body that transgresses boundaries, provides alternative meanings, and generates laughter, but it has little to do with an individual, autonomous subject.

Feces, Blood, and Other Pollutants

One important aspect of the grotesque body is its association with feces, urine, and other forms of filth. In tradition such materials are "gay matter," carnival substances related to the earth (Lachman 1988–89, 147). Bakhtin writes ([1968] 1984, 336), "As comic matter that can be interpreted bodily, [urine and dung] play an important part in . . . [grotesque] images. They appear in hyperbolic quantities and cosmic dimensions."

Physicians long have been concerned with feces and urine as part of medical practice. Patients that do not urinate or eliminate properly can be in grave danger, and so feces and urine are literally associated with life and death. In the excerpt that follows, neonatologist Dr. Massey talks about this fact: "One baby was going to die if she couldn't make urine. And so, she finally peed, and lived. And the dad was just screaming, 'I don't care! I'll change every diaper there ever was. I don't care if she pees all over the floor! I'm just so happy she's going to live.' And it just gives a lot of perspective to life" (Interview, November 5, 2019).

At the same time, physician concern with urine and excrement generates laughter and has done so since the medieval period. Marginalia from medieval manuscripts contain examples of parodic illustrations of animals impersonating physicians, who often hold a flask of urine called a "jordan" (Sprunger 1996). This is because the examination of urine, or "urinoscopy," was commonly used as a means of diagnosis. A border detail from the Metz Pontifical, for example, an early manuscript circa 1316, shows an ape examining a jordan while taking the pulse of his patient, who is either a stork or a crane. Medieval scholar David A. Sprunger (1996, 73) explains that apes were used for parodic purposes from the twelfth century onward and that apes and large wading birds often were depicted as being at odds, suggesting that the stork/crane in the illustration is ill-served by the physician-ape. Another example is an illustration in which a dog examines the jordan of a bedridden cat from a book of hours, dating from the second half of the fifteenth century. Dog and cats are traditional enemies, suggesting the patient is at the mercy of the physician (Sprunger 2016).

Parodies mocking associations between physicians, urine, and feces continued into the early modern period and beyond. The play Le Médecin Volant (1645), for example, by French playwright Molière (1622–1673) features a clownish servant sent to impersonate a doctor. The servant parodies medical education and techniques by "drink[ing] the urine sample with a little too much enthusiasm" (Livingston 1979, 679). Connections between physicians and excrement also are an aspect of Bakhtin's conception of the carnivalesque. Bakhtin ([1968] 1984, 161, 179) observes that Rabelais's "gay physician" was a paradoxical, ambivalent figure that combined elements of Hippocrates's noble physician with the image of a scatophagus (eater of excrement).

The example that follows is from *GomerBlog*. It illustrates the overlap between the practicalities of medical work and a carnivalesque orientation that conceives of excrement as gay matter associated with life. To contextualize the post, it must be understood that patients may not be allowed to leave the hospital until they have a bowel movement. Patients recovering from surgery in hospitals may be fine in all aspects and ready to go home, but they will not be discharged until there is a concrete sign that the bowels have "woken up" from anesthesia and are active. Physicians do not want patients in the hospital unnecessarily as hospital stays are expensive and take up resources, including valuable time. This is the underlying reason for the exuberance and joy (rather than mere juvenilism) manifested in the *GomerBlog* "Breaking News" article below (caps in original).

> THE PATIENT POOPED!!!.
> DURHAM, NC—HE POOPED!!!! OMG!!! Thank heavens! GomerBlog can't believe the news we're about to deliver! But he did it! HE DID IT!!! He pooped! The patient in room 423 at Durham Medical Center has POOPED! YeaahHHHHHH!!!! HERO STATUS Get the party hats, people!! Where are the funnel cakes, cupcakes?! Hire the mascots and the CLOWNS! FIREWORKS!!! Get the discharge paperwork ready and let the ticker-tape parades BEGIN! He has proved the doubters wrong! He sat upon his golden throne of white and delivered us a golden CHALICE filled with sensational stool!! Though pooped, he pooped! We must rejoice! In this Era of Constipation, we must always celebrate The Bowel Movement! ALWAYS!!! (Dr. 99 "Breaking News")

"Hyperbolic quantities" of feces here appear stylistically through the excessive use of capitalization and exclamation marks, exaggeration that Bakhtin observes is a typical indicator of the grotesque body.

The character Fats in Shem's *The House of God* can be interpreted as a carnivalesque character, as he is not bothered by excrement. He appropriately seeks to specialize in gastroenterology. Someone who chooses to be a gastroenterologist makes that decision partly on the fact that feces do not bother them a lot.

As Dr. Sheppard posited: "The question in choosing your specialty is: What is your limiting factor? Is it respiratory secretions? Then don't become a pulmonologist. Do dead bodies gross you out? Then don't do pathology. Do burn victims? Then don't do derm" (interview, September 20, 2019). This concept of one's "limiting factor" is the basis of another *GomerBlog* (n.d.) headline: "Graduating Colorectal Fellow Realizes She Hates Poop."

For Fats, stool is not a source of disgust but of wealth. Fats states bluntly: "There's a lotta money in shit" (Shem [1978] 2003, 33). Physicians in the hospital where Fats works make money by ordering unnecessary gastrointestinal workups. In the example that follows, Fats responds to a question about this unnecessary workup from his intern Potts:

> "What is it with this GI workup?" I asked. "She says she's depressed and has a headache."
>
> "It's the specialty of the House," said Fats, "the bowel run. TTB—Therapeutic Trial of Barium."
>
> "There's nothing therapeutic about barium. It's inert."
>
> "Of course it is. But the bowel run is the great equalizer."
>
> "She's depressed. There's nothing wrong with her bowels."
>
> "Of course there's not. There's nothing wrong with her, either." (33)

Fats goes on to point out that the new wing of the hospital is being built explicitly to conduct "bowel run[s] of the rich" (33).

The fact that Fats orders an unnecessary bowel procedure also links him to long-standing ideas about bogus medicine conducted solely for profit. Ancient forms of the carnivalesque were directly tied to the medicinal cries of mountebanks, druggists, and charlatans in the marketplace (see chap. 5). Bakhtin ([1968] 1984, 161) states that "mock prescriptions are one of the most widespread genres of grotesque realism." Significantly, however, Fats points out that his own "mock prescription" does actually help his patient feel better even though "nothing" is wrong with her. He is doing his job as a physician.

Excrement and urine also are connected to the grotesque body because they are associated with degradation. To "degrade" or "debase" means to lower, and the grotesque body degrades that which is official, esteemed, and exalted by society (such as values, ideas, people) by thrusting those elements of society into the bodily lower material stratum and mixing them with excrement, digestion, the bowels, or the genitalia. In doing so, a carnivalesque topsy-turveyness temporarily is achieved as the existing social order is refashioned by associating it with the lower stratum's alternative meanings. The idea is that the old, powerful, and established elements of society are reduced (degraded) to make room for new forms of social relations. For example, excrement or urine can be used to degrade by literally throwing feces on a person or object and thus covering that person or object in the meanings associated with shit. A classic example of degradation in Rabelais occurs when the giant Gargantua uses various objects to wipe himself and in the process "besmirches" them:

> Once I mopped my scut with the velvet scarf of a damozel. It was pleasurable: the soft material proved voluptuous and gratifying to my hindsight. Once, too, I used a hood, from the same source and with the same results. The next time it was her neckerchief; again, her crimson satin earpieces, but they were bespangled and begilt with beshitten jewelry that scraped my tailpiece from end to end.... Next, spirting behind a bush, I came upon a March cat.... and I put it to excellent advantage though its claws mildly lacerated my perinaeum. (Bakhtin [1968] 1984, 371)

Degradation is one of the most important ways that the grotesque body challenges officialdom, but degradation is difficult to contextualize because it has so many negative connotations. It is part of a comic mode known as *bathos*, in which something grand, lofty, or sacred is suddenly made vulgar. In the previous example, objects associated with feminine wealth and nobility, such as a neckerchief, velvet scarf, and fine jewelry, are made vulgar by their use. Degradation is more commonly accomplished at the symbolic level, for example by calling someone a polluting insult such as "shithead." Degradation may be accompanied by carnivalesque laughter, which also contributes to the upending of power. Through degradation, objects are accorded new meanings.

Excrement and urine are used for degradation because they are pollutants and, as discussed in chapter 3, pollutants delineate cultural boundaries. Society is built on cultural boundaries such as distinctions between self/other, cleanliness/filth, and order/chaos (Douglas [1966] 2003), and pollutants exist on the negative side of such divisions. In the aforementioned binaries, pollutants are associated with other, filth, and chaos, rather than self, cleanliness, and order. When something becomes associated with a pollutant, it also becomes associated with the negative side of foundational cultural categories (Douglas [1966] 2003). To be associated with a pollutant is to be degraded, to be transformed from an ordinary or valued set of meanings into a set of negative ones, meanings that threaten the established social order and thus serve carnivalesque purposes. This is why pollutants are ambivalent and dangerous, often hemmed in by taboo and ritual.

This means that the bodily substances with which care providers routinely work such as urine, blood, and feces are arenas of dense symbolic meaning.

Folklorist Kathleen Odean (1995, 137) in a fitting tribute to Freudian folklorist Alan Dundes once quipped that "anal folklore pervades the medical world," meaning that references to the bottom and to excrement permeate medical folklore. The stories, jokes, quips, proverbs, and sayings about bodily secretions that exist in medicine constitute a body of folklore that manage dirt.

The term "code brown," which parodies the hospital code system that assigns color codes to different types of emergencies, is one example. One humorous use of a code brown applies to physicians themselves, referring to a patient case that is so bad (meaning traumatic or stressful) that the doctor is shitting their pants. In *The House of God*, for example, the intern Potts is "so scared at the thought of seeing patients that I had an attack of diarrhea" (Shem [1978] 2003, 31) and hides out in the bathroom. The physician is debased: the conventional meanings surrounding the physician as assured, competent, and all knowing are transformed through a verbal association with their own excrement into someone who is incompetent, terrified, and has lost control of their (medicalized and professionalized) body.

Code browns can also be literal rather than metaphorical. Dr. Brian Goldman (2014, 44) writes that a "code brown" also is "known almost universally as slang for a patient poop emergency," meaning that a patient has lost control of their body and is having a severe case of diarrhea. Goldman pointedly notes that nurses—much more than doctors—have to clean up messes left by patients, and so they recall code brown cases in more detail. Physicians, however, also deal with patient excrement because they do the procedures to manage it. Such procedures violate boundaries, are degrading to both patient and physician, and evoke the grotesque body. One example is a procedure to relieve severe constipation. An endoscope is inserted into the anus to unblock the sigmoid colon, and a tube is then inserted through the scope. Once the tube hits the blockage, the blockage comes out as the intestine is decompressed. Goldman recounts a story in which this procedure was done before a bag was properly in place to catch the stool. The storyteller explains: "There was like a 'ping,' and the stool shot across the room and hit the curtain. The senior resident actually had to jump out of the way so as to not be hit with this high-velocity stool flying across the room. It was hysterical to us, but you have to try and maintain some professionalism" (46). The uncomfortable situation generates hilarity because the unmanaged dirt has debased the conventional meanings of the sterile and professional medical environment.

Another infamous way to relive severe or debilitating constipation (often a side effect of medication) is the manual fecal disimpaction procedure. Colloquially known as "scooping for poop" or "bobbing for apples," the manual fecal disimpaction procedure is an example of "scut work" (itself a scatological term)—that is, demeaning (debasing) work that physicians who are low on the medical hierarchy must sometimes do; the procedure of course also is debasing for the patient. It involves inserting a lubricated, gloved finger into the patient's rectum, breaking up the hardened stool using a scissoring motion, and using a hooked finger to remove it. The procedure is described in *The House of God* and is done by Fats and another resident named Teddy: "Double-gloved and surgically masked to filter out the smell, Teddy and Fats were digging at the endless stream of feces in Max's megacolon . . . From Teddy's radio poured Brahms. The smell was overpoweringly fresh shit" (Shem [1978] 2003, 267). This procedure, like massaging a human heart by hand previously described, is unimaginable to the general public but is an excellent example of how medical work is transgressive. It illustrates why the metaphorical concept of the grotesque body, a body that is transgressive, polluting, and boundary breaking, appears in medicine.

Scatological references are also found in formal jokes and proverbial sayings. Fat's bogus "trial of barium" is similar to the absurd and unnecessary medical procedure ("mock prescription") outlined in the following joke:

> There are only two reasons not to do a rectal exam:
> (1) the patient has no rectum and
> (2) the intern has no finger. (Odean 1995, 138)

An example of a scatological proverbial saying is the phrase "shit rolls downhill," which is an invective against medical hierarchies. It means that the lower on the medical hierarchy one is, the more likely one is to encounter terrible working conditions (including having to do scut work). Another example is "BOHICA" (bend over here it comes again) (Odean 1995), which compares terrible working conditions that one cannot avoid to unwanted anal sex.

Scatological terms of abuse or insults may be directed toward both patients and coworkers. These tend to be used mostly during the training period and have been amply documented (e.g., George and Dundes 1978; Gordon 1983; Odean 1995; Dans 2002; Winick 2004). Scholars interpret the use of terms such as *crock* (short for "crock of shit") as arising from stress, expressing hostility, and providing a sense of in-group solidarity. "Crock" was first documented by sociologist Howard S. Becker and colleagues (1961, 317), and it remained in use through the late twentieth century (see Becker 1993). Folklorist Stephen Winick (2004) argues that because filth goes against the established order, scatological terms of abuse were applied to patients who evaded categories, challenged hospital norms, and defied the established order by squandering time and resources. He writes that while such insults seem unethical, they paradoxically are rooted in a strong sense of ethics in which physicians desire to care for patients but resent patients who demand care and will not allow themselves to be cared for. He concludes, "It is the stress from *loss of control* that ultimately produces the filth metaphor" (100; italics mine).

Terms of abuse can be situated within the logic of a carnivalesque framework because terms of abuse invoke the wider aesthetic of the grotesque body. Insults, oaths, curses, and terms of abuse are part of what Bakhtin calls filthy and impertinent marketplace language that emerges not only in actual marketplaces but also anywhere people come together in familiar environments. Such speech is filled with rough bodily images, exists entirely outside official norms, refuses to conform to formal etiquette, and purposefully breaches the establishment (Bakhtin [1968] 1984, 145, 187, 319). Terms of abuse, curses, and oaths are antistructural, meaning that they generate new, alternative meanings in contradistinction to the official sanctioned order, and so abuse is a profoundly ambivalent act.

Even understood within a framework that invokes the grotesque body, however, slurs against patients are problematic due to issues of significant power differentials. Today insults against patients rarely are tolerated: physicians do not approve of calling patients names. The official stance of organized medicine is that the health and welfare of one's patients must be the physician's highest priority. From the viewpoint of the medical establishment, physicians should always act from a position of tolerance, respect, and service toward them, even if those patients are difficult, irrational, abusive, do not listen to medical advice, and take up a lot of time—the kinds of antistructural patients Winick identifies as being targets. Terms of abuse invert that official stance. On the other hand, physicians have power and patients have less, so while these examples invoke the grotesque body, they also reinforce existing hierarchies. It is easy to romanticize the carnivalesque as consisting of an inverted dynamic in which official power is lampooned, but this is not always the case. Historically, in addition to the elite, people without power, such as transgressive women, Jews, and other marginalized peoples, were targeted during pre-Lenten Carnival celebrations. No one was exempt from becoming a target and so carnival was particularly dangerous for such persons. That the weak and marginalized are also targeted means that that carnival can be vicious and cruel (Eagleton 2019a). Here the carnivalesque does not challenge official norms but reinforces them.

Physicians encounter other types of pollutants apart from feces and urine. Most doctors have personal experience narratives in which the physician, as a representative of the established medical order, ends up covered in blood, vomit, spittle, respiratory secretions, or vaginal fluids. Doctors are expected to behave in a professional, unemotional, and controlled (that is, medicalized) manner when such violations occur, but the reality is that degradation evokes laughter, even if the incident itself is not side-splittingly "funny." Dr. Adam Kay (2017, 41–42), for example, recounted during his ob-gyn residency in the UK in the early 2000s that "it's the third time in a week my boxers have been soaked in someone else's blood and I've had no option but to chuck them away and continue the shift commando." As another example, the following narrative was told to me by Dr. Warner in an interview conducted in 2020.

> So, as a medical student I had—I was operating with a surgeon who was a vascular surgeon. And I hadn't operated with him before, but when I had downtime, I'd go find someone that would let me operate with them. And I had put on some safety glasses (which was good), and he was sewing in a vascular graft.
>
> In fact, this type of thing happened to me twice, through all the years [laughs].
>
> But when you do vascular surgery, you have to clamp the artery, so that you don't have massive blood loss. So, time is of the essence, you want to restore blood flow as quickly as you can. So, it's a series of clamps: you clamp before, and you clamp after the area that you're going to put this graft on. And then you make an incision in the artery, and you sew this graft to it, and then you have to clamp the graft also, because when you open up the artery, it's going to fill the graft.
>
> And so, often you'll check to make sure that you have blood flow, by un-clamping the graft, or unclamping the artery. And you check for leaks around the graft by unclamping the artery and keeping the graft clamped. And so, this particular day, he unclamped the graft, and it just shot a stream of blood and hit me square in the forehead.
>
> And then was just dripping down my nose, inside of my safety glasses. I was very grateful I'd put [laughs] glasses on that day, because I often (at that point) did not wear safety glasses. . . . And he just kept—he didn't know he did it. And finally, after a couple of minutes—and this is just dripping down my face—one of the nurses stopped him and said, "Do you mind if we wipe his face off?" And he looks up, and he's like, "Oh, sorry. That's fine. Hurry." (Interview, January 13, 2020)

The medical student could not touch his own face to wipe off the blood. Once a physician has been made sterile through a series of ritualistic steps, they are forbidden to break the sterile field by touching anything inside it. The student was unable to do anything to stop the blood from dripping down his face. The nonchalant response of the attending surgeon is part of the comedy; his response to the dripping blood is to focus on the job at hand: "That's fine. Hurry."

The previous narrative quickly led to a similar follow-up story by Dr. Warner:

> It happened again, as a resident—where I was helping a vascular surgeon (this was later on in my residency, so I was more involved in this case). And he was doing, it's called a fem-fem bypass—which is (I don't even know if they do these much anymore, because surgeries change so much)—so anyway, you graft from the femoral artery on one side (on the right side, in this case) to the femoral artery on the left side, because they have a blockage in their iliac artery. So, you're bypassing all the blockage and sending blood down the leg.
>
> And this surgeon had the graft kind of hanging off the edge of the table and forgot to clamp it, and I didn't notice it. And as we were working, he was unclamping it, and checking everything. And after twenty or thirty seconds, I just had this warm sensation on my foot. And I looked down, and it was just draining straight down my leg and into my shoe.
>
> It just filled my shoe with blood. And so, I just said, "You might want to clamp this; I think you need to clamp this." (Interview, January 13, 2020)

In both narratives, the patient body is a grotesque body: it has erupted beyond its own boundaries and fused with the outside world. The result for the student, who represents official organized medicine and culture, is pollution and degradation, the emergence of new meanings, and the generation of laughter, at least after the fact.

The next story also is about the unexpected eruption of bodily fluids. It is about a practical joke that was played by a forensic pathologist on a student when she was doing premed volunteer work at the local coroner's office.

> One of the forensic pathologists, he was probably in his seventies at the time and he'd been doing this his whole career. They don't retire until they die themselves basically. And, there was a body that we were working on and the stomach was superprotruded. It was a male, but the body looked like it was pregnant. It was huge, huge, huge, and it was my job to do the first cut, that Y incision. And I was like "what is in that belly?" because it was really taut and hard. And he was like, "Oh this guy just had cancer, don't worry, you are going to open it and you are going to see a big tumor." And I was like "OK," you know?—whatever, he's been doing this for decades

and decades. So I did the Y incision and when I got to the bottom of the sternum to get into the abdominal cavity, greenish, yellowish fluid flew over the dead body's head, and onto the floor, and soaked me head to toe. And the forensic pathologist I was working with was laughing so hard tears were streaming down his face. Because he knew exactly what was in there! He knew it was going to happen, totally. He totally knew. And I'm covered in grossness. Luckily we are completely geared up. I didn't get it on any of my actual clothes or on my skin or anything like that—he would never put me in harm's way—but it was gross. That was probably one of the grossest things I've ever experienced in my life. [Laughs.] (Anonymous, interview, June 13, 2020)

Here the grotesque body again erupts beyond itself; that the student is covered in pollutants and degraded is obvious. The threat to cultural categories is seen as funny, eliciting laughter on the part of the forensic pathologist. He played a practical joke, which functions to initiate the student into a group (Marsh 2015).

The final narrative example was told to me by a friend. The ob-gyn who did her delivery ended up covered in amniotic fluid and her regular ob-gyn later told her about the joking exchange between the two physicians afterward. My friend was the patient.

I had preeclampsia and pregnancy-induced high blood pressure with my first pregnancy and had to be induced, so my ob-gyn was watching my second pregnancy closely for signs of high blood pressure. When I was near my due date, he offered to strip my membranes so that I would go into labor before my blood pressure climbed too high. I didn't go into labor that weekend, but then on Monday morning, I woke up with contractions. The contractions were very irregular and impossible to time, and I realized the baby was coming fast. We live only about five miles from the hospital, but by the time we arrived at the hospital, I was already dilated to ten [centimeters] and the baby's head was visible. I remember stripping off my clothes and throwing myself naked on the table, ready to push that baby out. The nurse told me not to push, and she ran to get a doctor—there was no time to call my ob-gyn, but luckily there was an ob-gyn in the hospital who was waiting the required time after delivering a baby by VBAC [vaginal birth after cesarean section]. He came into the room and told me to push really hard because according to the fetal monitor, the baby was in distress (it turns out there was a true knot in the cord). I pushed really hard and my water burst—all over the doctor! I remember he was wearing glasses but no other protective gear—basically my water squirted out all over him! To top it off, the baby had pooped in the womb and my amniotic fluid was FULL of poo, which got all over him too! It was a mess.

Anyway, my baby ended up in the NICU for a few days, and I remember that when I finally brought her to my regular ob-gyn's office for an appointment, he told me that he got the ob-gyn who delivered her a gift. He said usually he got docs who delivered his babies a gift certificate for dinner at a nice restaurant, but he said in my case, it was more fitting to send him a gift certificate for a car wash. We both had a good laugh over that one! (Personal communication sent by email, February 10, 2010)

Pregnancy and birth are intimately associated with the grotesque body. Cultural theorist Mary Russo (1986) illustrated that the grotesque body can be read as inherently female. The grotesque body is in the process of becoming, fusing with the outside world and dissolving into other bodies, and this is nowhere more obvious than during birth. In this story, the pregnant patient's body discharges in unexpected ways. It is expected that the mother's water will break but not all over the physician. Further, this amniotic fluid was particularly polluting since it was filled with meconium. The crux of the story, however, is the surprise gift certificate. The certificate implies that the delivering physician needed to be cleaned on a grand scale—the scale of a car. The certificate suggests the "bigness" of the event: the birth, the mother's pregnant body, and the gush of polluted water that warranted an entire car wash rather than simply, say, a shower.

Gigantism

Another important aspect of the grotesque body is gigantism and the association between gigantism and eating and drinking. The central characters in Rabelais's writings are two giants named Pantagruel and Gargantua. The antics of these giants, their huge bodies, and their enormous appetites (for food, sex, violence) are the basis of the grotesque, which, as explained previously, is intimately connected to images of the mouth, the act of swallowing, the belly, the digestive system, and birth. In Rabelais's hyperbolic explanation of the origins of people, for example, he uses images of giants. He writes that after Cain slew Abel, the earth became extraordinarily fertile and medlars grew extremely large. The people who ate medlars (a fruit similar to a date) then grew to gigantic proportions. There were men with monstrous bellies, as well as abnormally large noses and ears, and men with disproportionately large phalluses and testes (in Morris 1994, 165–67).

The gigantic body contrasts with the normative medical body. If the ideal-ized medicalized body is contained and controlled, the gigantic one is not. Scholarship on fatness concludes that while meanings of the fat body have changed over time and are historically contingent, fatness generally is under-stood as both unruly and transgressive. The gigantic body is one that literally spills over itself and refuses to be contained within "proper" boundaries, which is why eating and drinking (gluttony) are associated with it.

The character Fats, for example, is carnivalesque not only because of his association with excrement but also because of his large physical size and ap-petite. Most obviously, his nickname is "Fats" or "the Fatman." He has a number of bellies and chins, and he is known for his prodigious appetite in addition to his medical expertise. In the novel, the protagonist Potts describes Fats as "the one best at eating, best at medicine, my resident, the Fat Man. The Fat Man shoveling onions and Hebrew National hot dogs and raspberry ice cream into his mouth all at once at the ten-o'clock supper" (Shem [1978] 2003, 4–5). Potts also observes, "The Fat Man had strict priorities, and at the top was food. Until that awesome tank of a mind had been fueled via that eager nozzle of a mouth, Fats had low tolerance for medicine, academic or otherwise, and for anything else" (30).

The Fat Man also is respected. Potts states, "He was wonderful and a wonder. Brooklyn-born, New York City-trained, expansive, impervious, brilliant, effi-cient, from his sleek black hair and sharp black eyes and bulging chins through his enormous middle that forced his belt buckle to roll over on its belly like a shiny fish, to his wide black shoes, the Fat Man was fantastic" (Shem [1978] 2003, 26). Fats is known for his personality, kindness, and hope that he gives to the new interns; these meanings hearken to older, more positive notions of the gigantic body as associated with abundance and life. Not surprisingly Fats also is associated with laughter: "Fats burst into laughter. Big juicy laughs rolled down from his eyes to his cheeks to his chins to his bellies" (47).

One example of the gigantic body in medicine comes in the form of morbidly obese patients, who may become objects of talk. Informal talk about obesity exists but is difficult to document. None of the physicians I interviewed talked about morbid obesity, and I did not pursue this line of questioning. The reason such talk exists is that physicians deal with all kinds of bodies, but severely obese patients tend to have more health problems, challenging normative ide-als. For example, extreme obesity often leads to an early death and complicates surgery. There are higher rates of diabetes and higher rates of infection. Mor-bidly obese patients also may require special medical equipment as they may not fit into regular machinery, such as an MRI. In her description of a kidney transplant performed on an obese patient, Young (1997, 90) explains, "Fat people are harder to operate on than thin ones. The layer of fat just under the skin is itself delicate: it bleeds easily and is difficult to sew up. But the width of the fat layer also increases the depth of the hole in which the surgical team must operate, through which they must pass to get to the kidney. On Ms. Brown, this layer is a handspan across. But the fat also greases the instruments, the gloves, the suture material, and the vessels making fine vascular procedures like this one more difficult to perform." Indeed, surgeons are the medical specialty stereotyped for sometimes making comments about severely obese patients.

Like other aspects of the grotesque body such as abuse and filth, fatness is coded negatively in modern social thought. Many of the traditional positive meanings associated with fatness such as life, generosity, laughter, and abundance no longer inhere or are quite buried. Instead fatness today is associated with negative traits such as lack of control or a lack of willpower. Fat people may be seen as greedy and lazy. Fatness is also enmeshed in modern discourses of health and ideologies regarding self-control, individual responsibility, and morality: an overweight body often is seen as self-indulgent and immoral (Lupton 2003, 43). Thus unlike cancer patients for example, morbidly obese people may be held responsible both by physicians and the general public for their own condition.

Fat also is largely coded as female. Russo (1986) observed similarities between the grotesque body and the feminine, suggesting that it is really femaleness that threatens the established order. The fat female body signifies hunger for both food and sex, challenging patriarchal norms that dictate women should be controlled (Zimdars 2015). Obese men also may be coded as female: they may be viewed as effeminate and therefore presumed to be weak. Media theorists Anne Graefer, Allaina Kilby, and Inger-Lise Kalviknes Bore (2019), for example, examined carnivalesque images of Donald Trump's body as it was depicted on protest signs during the January 2018 Women's March. These images depicted Trump's body as fat and orange with tiny hands / small penis. They observed that while such images were carnivalesque in that they targeted power and focused on a fat, transgressive body, they also were conservative as they "confirm normative assumptions about White masculinity" (172). Both fat women and fat men are seen as needing to be brought under control as part of what Angela Stukator (2001, 203) calls "reactionary body politics."

Young (1997, 90) documents an example of a fat comment between surgeons during the kidney transplant: "In the course of surgery, Henry Scott, the surgeon who is opening up the recipient in the adjoining operating room at the same time that Adam Tartakoff is taking the kidney out of the donor, comes in to see how far along his colleague has gotten. Dr. Tartakoff says, 'Hi, Henry. This lady had a one-legged sea captain strapped to her side and we had just a little trouble getting him off.' Dr. Scott replies, 'That is a gigantic hole. What is up there, the heart?'" Young observes, "Allusion, however witty, to the woman as a whale attests to her objectification. In the first instance, it emphasizes her solidity. She is reduced to her heft. In the second, it elides her personhood. Such a remark would never be made in her presence. It presumes an absence" (90). In other words, there is no individual with a personhood during surgery, and the body is treated as an object. This absence allows both the surgery to occur and the emergence of the comment.[5] The follow-up comment referencing "the giant hole" has less to do with the patient's obesity than with jesting competitiveness between the surgeons. Dr. Scott teases Dr. Tartakoff about the size of the surgical hole he has made (presumably because of the patient's large size), thereby jokingly questioning the surgeon's competency (see chap. 5).

The oblique reference to obese persons as whales is not limited to Young's example. Dr. Brian Goldman has an entire chapter in his book called "harpooning the whale" in which he documents medical folk terms for obesity. Some of his terms came from anesthesiologists because severe obesity can make it difficult to insert needles to administer drugs. For extremely obese patients needing an epidural, for example, anesthesiologists use an extralong Tuohy needle to insert an epidural catheter, a needle that was developed specifically to accommodate extra layers of tissue in the back (Goldman 2014, 190). This needle and the procedure led to the name of the title of Goldman's chapter.

Comments on fatness mediate the dynamics of discipline and carnival: they acknowledge the transgressiveness of fat bodies in the service of medicalized ideals. They are another example of how a carnivalesque orientation can target the always already marginalized and reinforce power differentials. This also is true for fatness in modern comedy generally, where fatness is spectacle and exploited as a form of otherness. Stukator (2001, 202) writes, "In contemporary mainstream comedy, the spectacle of the fat woman epitomizes Bakhtin's grotesque body and its functions as a symbol of ambivalence. She is constructed as disgusting and delightful, attractive and repulsive, normal and deviant. Yet that initial ambivalence is invariably replaced and resolved by hegemonic certainties" (for an exception, see Zimdars 2015). This dynamic is similar in medicine, which acknowledges the transgressiveness and ambivalence of gigantism but ultimately seeks to control and contain it within "hegemonic certainties."

One example of talk about patients that closely hews to traditional notions of giants is the comparison of patients on one's service to "rocks" and "boulders." In folklore, giants are closely related to the landscape. Legends in Scandinavia, for example, frequently connect giants to landscape formations, including large rocks (Kvideland and Sehmsdorf 1988). Bakhtin ([1968] 1984, 328) writes, "The giants and their legends are closely related to the grotesque conception of the body. . . . Most local legends connect such natural phenomena as mountains, rivers, rocks, and islands with the bodies of giants or with their different organs; these bodies are, therefore, not separated from the world or from nature." In medical parlance, "rocks" and "boulders" are patients on a hospital service who cannot be transferred to another service and are too sick to be discharged from the hospital.[6] They are called "rocks" because they are difficult to move anywhere else and so remain on one's service for a long period of time. Doctors with a lot of rocks on their service might be known as "rock collectors" or as having "rock gardens." "How's the rock garden?" is a question these caregivers might be asked. Particularly obese patients who can't be moved off one's service might be referred to as "boulders," and so in this example, the gigantic body becomes part of the hospital's landscape.

In sum, morbid obesity, as a signifier of giantism, challenges the idealized, controlled medical body. The folklore that exists in medicine surrounding extreme fatness acknowledges the gigantic body as unruly, uncontained, and transgressive, supporting the claim that a latent concept of the grotesque body occurs in medicine. Such comments also illustrate that the carnivalesque is not always funny and does not always upend power but rather may target the weak and/or marginalized to reinforce norms. Physician comments on fatness therefore discipline in the service of the status quo while acknowledging the existence of transgressive and ambivalent bodies, bodies that both reinforce and challenge dominant truths by their very existence.

Dismemberment

A final way in which the grotesque body manifests in medicine is through dismemberment, in which the interior becomes visible. This is why a carnivalesque orientation emerges in gross anatomy (see chap. 3). Stories about bodily trauma permeate medical practice. The story that follows is from my father-in-law's repertoire. He told me about a patient who had been living with part of an ice pick in his skull for several decades.

> **LG:** One of my favorite stories is where you talk about the guy with the pickax.[7]
> **WW:** With the pick in his head?
> **LG:** Yeah, can you tell that story?

WW: Actually, I actually saw that at St. Vincent's Hospital: where a fellow came in with something—he got a head X-ray, and there's a pick inside his skull, inside his brain. And trying to get a history of what might have happened. He said, "Well some guy did come at me with an ice pick about twenty years ago. But I thought he missed."

LG: [Laughing.]

WW: But obviously, he didn't. (Walsh, interview, December 2, 2012)

This tale is narratable because of the central amazing fact: a man unknowingly had lived for years with an ice pick embedded in his skull. The final line provides the coda and evaluation: "I thought he [the opponent] missed." The line is comic because the opponent clearly did not, and so the story is about a living body that should be dead. Such tales illustrate how bodies stretch the boundaries of imagination and believability yet are grounded in the actual events of physician work.

Emergency room physicians commonly encounter physical trauma. Such stories can be horrific, but more often they are both terrible and comic because the events and bodies expand conceptions of the ordinary. Pediatric emergency doctor Maija Elonen explained that she loved working with kids because, despite the horrible things that occurred, the kids themselves were "awesome." In her stories, the focus was on the incongruity between the child's injured body, the strange or bizarre situation, and the cheerful, even exuberant attitude of the kids, whom, she noted, were "all good" once the acute injury or illness was resolved.

ME: So, when kids are well, they're well, right? They're pretty funny when they turn around. And sometimes, just a little bit of Tylenol or Motrin turns them from lethargic, to totally well. Or sometimes their stories are pretty funny: how they come in and [laughs] get themselves into different binds, you know?

We've had a kid—he put his finger in one of these washers that was attached to a bike. And so, he came in with his finger stuck to basically a bike And we were trying to figure out, "Okay, how are we going to saw this off?" You know, "We need to get some serious equipment from Lowe's in order to figure this out."

[Laughter.]

And here is this kid, you know? And you're like, "How did that happen?"

I had another kid that was in a bike accident, and somehow—I have no idea, but somehow got the handlebar literally sticking through his leg. And…somebody was able to disconnect the handlebar from the bike;

but you know, they're sitting there. And they're fine, because the pain is controlled with morphine. But they're just sitting there and they're like, "I don't know how this happened." [Laughing.] And here they are, with a bike handle through their whole femur.

LG: Right.

ME: They just get themselves into binds. Sometimes you're just like, "How did this happen?"

LG: "How did you do that?"

ME: [Laughs.] Because they are all in, right? (Interview, June 19, 2020)

In contrast to the terrible injury (a bicycle handlebar sticking out of the femur, a finger stuck in a bike), the children were not in severe pain. Instead they were full of life and excitement, providing a comic effect. The physicians also are rendered comical, transformed into common mechanical workers who must remove bike parts with tools obtained at Lowe's.

Sometimes the stories highlighted the stupidity that led to the injury. One surgeon I interviewed told me about a patient who shot off his hand by pulling a loaded rifle, muzzle first, toward him through a fence. The trigger caught on the fence, and the gun went off, blowing off the patient's fingers. The surgeon was tasked with reconstructing the hand.

Surgery is the arena in which the body is opened and internal organs are exposed, and so arguably surgery itself engages the grotesque body. Dr. Warner stated that he simply liked "playing in people's guts."

IW: I still like getting my hands in the belly. There's a tactile sensation, and there's a smell—

LG: Um-hmm?

IW: And it's weird to say, but you just get this flood of senses when you have someone's abdomen open and you're playing with their intestines. [Laughs.]

LG: Huh.

IW: I shouldn't say "playing" I guess, but—

LG: It's a little bit like playing.

IW: I think it is, when you enjoy what you do.

LG: Yeah.

IW: It's all playing. (Interview, January 13, 2020)

Tales of dismemberment are not limited to physicians. First responders such as EMTs tell graphic stories about horrific scenes they encounter. Tim

Tangherlini notes, however, that most were not told for ghoulishness but for the bizarreness of the situation. He also intimates the underlying idea of an ambivalent, grotesque body that elicits laughter. One of his informants recounted a story in which the person was clearly dead, but the hospital physicians tried to save him anyway, resulting in a morbid treatment of the corpse. Tangherlini (1998, 56) writes, "The [unnecessary] medical treatment approaches the grotesque, since the patient is so clearly dead. But in Lars' [the narrator's] capable narrative hands, the story does not devolve into a depressing rumination on the horrors of the assault and the ghoulish attempts to revive the patient; instead, he turns it into a burlesque." Tangherlini does not mean *grotesque* in the sense I use it here, but his combination of the terms *grotesque* and *burlesque* invokes a sense of the grotesque, carnivalesque body. Tangherlini concludes, "In his story he [Lars] ultimately recognizes that life—and death—are unpredictable and that all one can do, when confronted with these contractions, is laugh" (67).

Conclusion

The folklore about the body that physicians tell can easily seem horrific, insensitive, callous, juvenile, or just plain gross. But such stories are not intended for outsiders: the audience is other doctors or caregivers who work intimately with the body on a daily basis and who risk defilement by doing so.

The reason talk about the body might seem gross, horrific, or insensitive is that modern audiences labor under modern conceptions of the body. Modern conceptions of the body idealize the body as private, individualized, closed, controlled, and contained and in which binaries such as life and death are separated. This idealized conception of the body also exists in medicine; indeed, the medical world produced this conception of the body and strives to reproduce it.

Body-oriented stories and talk do not subvert this idealized norm—they reinforce it—but they acknowledge the existence of a different kind of body, the grotesque body, a body that not only is transgressive but that also actually reflects real people and the realities of medical work. The idealized medicalized body is the goal, but that is not the body with which physicians work. As Bakhtin ([1968] 1984, 179) observes, "The physician [in tradition] ... is not concerned with a completed and closed body but with the one that is born, which is in the stage of becoming. The body that interests him is pregnant, delivers, defecates, is sick, dying, and dismembered. In one word, it is the body as it appears in abuses, curses, oaths, and generally in all grotesque images." This remains true in the modern world, where the ancient conception of a grotesque body remains useful for doctors as they navigate the realities of their work.

Notes

1. Doctors always acknowledge that individual pathology doesn't follow normal patterns; some individual pathology, however, may be quite aberrant and cause significant problems in surgery or treatment.

2. Modern scholarship frequently identifies technocratic techniques such as case studies as depersonalizing, but Foucault argues that medical and psychiatric techniques actually produced subjectivity in new ways and that these techniques are linked to the rise of the individual. For example, disciplinary power is concerned with the ever-finer and more highly grained applications of power and control; ideally, power is tailored to every individual and becomes internalized as the subject takes over the task of discipline themselves.

3. While there are many problems with western biomedical models, I am not antimedicine. My interest in describing this technical, authoritative, and reductionist approach is because it provides a framework for an oppositional perspective that entails the complex and expansive imagery of the grotesque body.

4. The biological body is the primary focus of most branches of medicine, and the basic systems of orientation in medicine do not address the patient as an individual person. Physicians-in-training study the body as individual compartmentalized systems with anatomical derivatives. Medical folklore mirrors this orientation.

5. This example underscores that individual subjects are not the focus of bodily oriented talk. As a comparison, university professors sometimes talk about poor, often funny, student writing: such talk is about the writing itself and usually not the student as a person. This perspective is not meant to be an apology but merely an observation.

6. See discussion of buffing and turfing in the introduction.

7. A pickax is how I remembered the story and so is how I identified the object in my interview question, but the object was an ice pick.

5

"I Need to Fix It"

Spurious and Expert Knowledge

And so, there's a pathologist, a psychiatrist, an internal medicine doc, and a surgeon [who] go duck hunting. And there's a bunch of birds fly[ing] over their hide, and one of them says, "Oh, look, look! Ducks."

And the internal medicine doctor says, "Well you know, they might not be ducks; there's a huge differential: they could be pigeons, they could be, you know, cormorants. Who knows what they could be: we really do need to exclude all the other possibilities before we really, definitively say they're ducks."

The psychiatrist says, "Well, you know, it doesn't really matter whether they are ducks or not; the important thing is whether they really realize that they are ducks. If they're at one with their duck-ness, then they truly are ducks; and if they're not, then they're not."

The surgeon just loads up and just blasts the shit out of them all.

And as they all fall to the ground, he turns to the pathologist and says, "Go find me a duck."

—Mark York, interview, September 6, 2018

One important target of the medical carnivalesque is medical knowledge and expertise. Doctors poke fun at what they know, what they don't know, and also what other doctors know and supposedly don't know. The joke that begins this chapter mocks medical expertise by drawing on esoteric stereotypes. Internal medicine physicians think specifically through all possibilities before making a diagnosis, and so in the joke the internist is hesitant to identify the bird as a duck. Psychiatrists accord primary importance to mental states, an orientation comically applied to ducks. Surgeons are caricatured as action-oriented, which results in an uncritical shooting. But the crux of the joke hinges on the relationship of surgeons to pathologists. Surgeons cut tissue and send it to pathology, while the pathologist determines what kind of tissue it is. It is pathologists, not surgeons, who make a final diagnosis and so in the joke the surgeon instructs the pathologist to "find me a duck" to justify the uncritical shooting-qua-surgery, a tagline that indexes the droll surgical mantra: "Sometimes wrong, but never uncertain."

Humor targeting medical knowledge and expertise also is found online. One example is the reference work *Gomerpedia*, described on the main web page on July 10, 2023, by its creators as "a woefully inaccurate medical encyclopedia for the modern medical professional. Please grab your books, dump them in the trash, apply ample amounts of lighter fluid, and set on fire."[1] *Gomerpedia* parodies the term *encyclopedia* by combining it with the slang term "gomer" (see George and Dundes 1978), which refers to an older patient who needs care but does not have a definable sickness. *Gomerpedia* is a nonsense word, the meaning of which is ambiguous but seems to signify a useless reference work.

Some entries for *Gomerpedia* poke fun at medical tools and techniques. Under the broad category of "medical devices," for example, one can find parodic entries for alleged medical instruments such as "pogo stick" and "duct tape" as well as the "da Vinci," an actual surgical system robot whose "utility is indirectly proportional to its cost." There also is an entry for a "large bore needle," which is immediately followed by an entry for a "large boar needle": "Used in emergency situations to deliver fluid or blood products quickly, a large boar needle is effective but terrifying since they can weigh up to 800 lbs." Another example is the "Amazon Electrocardiogram," a wireless cloud-connected machine that goes by the name Alyssa and that parodies Amazon's popular virtual assistant Alexa. Invented orders for the Amazon electrocardiogram include "Alyssa, what kind of heart attack am I having?" and "Alyssa, can you start chest compressions?" Other *Gomerpedia* entries parody medical terminology. The entry for "Healthcare System" contains no actual definition but rather says, "See *circus*," while the entry for "Referred Pain" reads: "Referred Pain is a type of pain patients experience when their primary care physician can't figure out a complaint and refers them to a subspecialist who doesn't have an appointment opening for at least 3 months." "Pain and suffering" is described as "a legal term for the physical and emotional stress that results from an injury. Medical providers often sue their patients for damages as a result of the depression and scarring," a tongue-in-cheek entry that alludes to the notion that taking care of people affects providers (see chap. 2). These examples illustrate that physicians mock themselves by targeting both their own expertise and the institution of medicine itself.

Doctors possess what Anthony Giddens (1990) calls "expert knowledge," which is highly technical expertise based on years of training. This kind of knowledge is not subject to verification and testing by lay people because it is too complicated or advanced, yet modern society relies on such expert knowledge to function. People who do not have expert knowledge must trust that the expertise of others is valid. Airline pilots are another example of a group that possesses expert knowledge. Lay people must trust and rely on their expertise in order to fly. "Spurious knowledge," in contrast, refers to knowledge or expertise that is suspect, sham, or potentially bogus. As I discuss in the section below, medicine has a long history of being suspected as "spurious knowledge," and only within the past hundred years or so has it fully become an authoritative discourse and realm of expert knowledge. Medicine in the past was suspect in part because of its associations with profit, theater, and the marketplace. Medical marketplace elements, such as mock prescriptions, miracle cures, and vendor's cries, are part and parcel of old forms of the carnivalesque. Folklore targeting medical specialties reanimates carnivalesque themes of doctors as incompetent, lazy, or arrogant, reframing medical knowledge as spurious, rather than expert. This mockery also temporarily undermines medical claims to truth and power, a characteristic of the carnivalesque.

The Historically Precarious Status of Academic Medical Knowledge

Medicine did not always have the aristocratic status it enjoys today. As noted in the introduction, the ridicule of academic medical knowledge (albeit not necessarily by physicians themselves) dates at least to the Middle Ages. Academic medicine in the Middle Ages lacked practical application, and physicians were lampooned as well-educated persons who were pompous, spoke nonsense, and were largely interested in status and money.

Comic ambivalence about physicians continued into the Renaissance. Dholakia, Friend, and Maguire (2016) call representations of physicians in Renaissance plays "figures of fun." The author notes that during the Renaissance, "We encounter doctors willing to make house calls to ladies' chambers for non-medical reasons; surgeons are satirized for their 'hard words,' and doctors for the frequency with which they prescribe laxatives. Shakespeare, too, offered stereotypes. In *Twelfth Night* when Sir Toby calls for a surgeon to treat his head wounds, he is told 'O, he's drunk, Sir Toby, an hour ago; his eyes were set at eight i' th' morning'" (Dholakia, Friend, and Maguire 2016, 1), meaning that when drunk, a person's eyes don't move, much like a dead person.[2]

Medicine was difficult to distinguish from showmanship and entertainment, particularly the theatrical popular entertainments found in the marketplace. Early modern literature and theater scholar M. A. Katritzky (2001, 122) writes that during the early modern period, "No firm lines can be drawn between the medical and cosmetic products peddled by mountebanks and those prescribed by qualified physicians." The term *mountebank* was first used in print in Europe in 1566 and is defined in the *Oxford English Dictionary* (*OED*) as "an itinerant charlatan who sold supposed medicines and remedies, frequently using various entertainments to attract a crowd of potential customers."[3] Similarly, a "charlatan" (first emerging in print in 1618 according to the *OED*) is described as a "a mountebank or Cheap Jack who descants volubly to a crowd in the street; *esp.* an itinerant vendor of medicines who thus puffs his 'science' and drugs."[4] Katritzky (2001, 121) writes that such persons combined the medicinal, the itinerant, and the theatrical.

The theatrical and marketplace elements of medicine were important aspects of Rabelais's carnivalesque. Vendors' cries, such as those found in Paris from sellers of medicine, were part of the popular-festive system of carnivalesque images. Bakhtin ([1968] 1984, 185) writes that "these tirades are one of the oldest practices of the market. The image of the physician advertising his remedy is also one of the oldest in world literature." This is because there existed "an ancient connection between the forms of medicine and folk art which explains the combination in one person of actor and druggist" (159). He additionally notes that Rabelais's novel is metamedical, as it takes on the language of the medical marketplace, promoting itself as a kind of literary cure in the carnivalesque tradition of mock prescriptions (161).

The physician as a combination of "actor and druggist" is perhaps why physicians became popular characters in theatrical performances. The stereotype of the inept, comic doctor reached theatrical heights in the stock comic character *Il Dottore*, the Doctor, which emerged on the stage in Italian commedia dell'arte in 1560 (Duchartre 1966, 196).[5] Commedia dell'arte characters were influenced by Carnival practices (Taviani 2018), and scholars characterize the Doctor specifically as a "gross Carnival figure" (Rudlin 1994, 99), directly connecting academic medicine and carnival. Il Dottore was supposedly from Bologna and therefore learned, since Bologna is home to one of the earliest European universities and is still a major medical school. Il Dottore was not always a physician, per se, but rather represented a university-educated person: he sometimes was a physician but could also represent a lawyer or scholar. Duchartre (1966, 200) explains that Il Dottore's typical costume in the sixteenth century was an exaggerated version of the black dress men of science and letters in Bologna. His

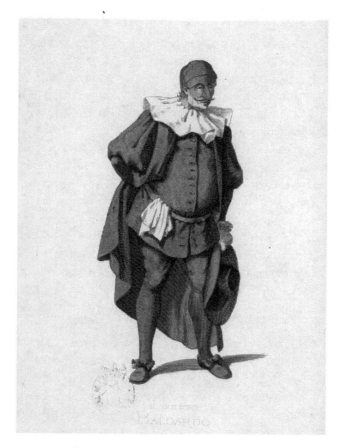

Figure 5.1. Illustration of *Il Dottore* by Maurice Sand.

theatrical mask covered the forehead and nose, while his cheeks were smeared with red. During some periods he also had a short, pointed beard (201) (see fig. 5.1). His large, bulbous nose represents drunkenness, and his large size is associated with gluttony.

One common name for the Doctor was Gracian Boloardo, *boloardo* meaning "dolt," and much of Il Dottore's hilarity came from his ridiculous or bizarre treatments and cures.[6] A main aspect of Il Dottore's character is that he spends his entire life "learning everything without understanding anything" (Duchartre 1966, 196). He speaks in non sequiturs or may quote Latin inaccurately, and his main comic character traits are ego, pride, and ineptitude. Duchartre describes him as "an eternal gas bag," and further notes that "he is endowed with prodigious aplomb, which usually intimidates even the best instructed of his listeners until, unable to endure any more, they rise up and give him a sound [carnivalesque] beating" (1966, 196).

Comic depictions of inept physicians continued in theater in the work of French playwright Molière (1622–1673), who was strongly influenced by Italian commedia dell'arte. His farces were concerned with medicine and consistently portrayed physicians as fools or a kind of clown (Livingston 1979). As philosopher Paisley Livingston (1979, 676) writes, "Indeed, Molière's doctors never cure anyone, and are permitted to remain on stage only long enough to demonstrate their vanity and total incompetence." The best-known example is *A Physician in Spite of Himself* (1666/1667), in which a lazy, drunken woodcutter presents himself as a doctor. He either speaks boastfully or speaks nonsense, and his cures are fake; however, his eccentricities are taken for brilliance, and he is sought out for his cures before eventually being discovered as an impostor.[7]

Medicine shows in the United States, which were popular in the 1800s, combined medical knowledge, showmanship, theater, and the marketplace. Medicine shows were traveling rural entertainments that merged pseudoscience, sales, advertising, and entertainment to sell patent medicines, such as tonics, liniments, and miracle elixirs to the public. The shows featured a "doctor" (i.e., a pitchman), who gave a medicine lecture in an overblown rhetorical style to audiences (McNamara 1984) and who sold medicine in between the entertainment acts. The formal entertainments included musical performances, dance, joke telling, ventriloquism, blackface, and other vaudeville performance styles. The medicines themselves, known as "patent medicines," were not medicines consisting of patented combinations of ingredients as understood today but rather were unregulated concoctions sold under a patented label (Kruesi 2004). The most famous of these was Clark Stanley's Snake Oil Liniment, which eventually earned sellers of patent medicines generic nicknames like "snake oil salesmen," meaning someone who sold worthless goods. Patent medicines emerged hand in hand with early forms of medical advertising found in almanacs and newspapers (Kruesi 2004). Often patent medicines didn't work, were potentially dangerous, or simply contained large amounts of alcohol or drugs like opium and THC, which presumably made them popular. Most medicine shows were sponsored by drug companies which sold their own exclusive patent medicines, making explicit the links between medicine, showmanship and entertainment, profit, and advertising. Although medicine shows largely were associated with the nineteenth century, they could still be found in the United States up through and even after World War II (Wagner and Zeitlin 1983).

Formal medical training in the US also was unregulated and associated with advertising and profit until the early twentieth century. With the notable exception of John Hopkins, most medical schools were private, for-profit nonacademic institutions. Student learning was ad hoc, unstandardized, and frequently inadequate. Students who wanted a complete medical education went to study in Europe. The situation was so bad that in 1910 the Carnegie Foundation commissioned the Flexner report, which surveyed the state of medical education in the United States and Canada. The report scathingly critiqued the majority of existing institutions, noting that "for the most part they can be called schools or institutions only by courtesy" (Flexner 1910, 6). Noting the long-standing link between medicine and advertising, the report's author, Abraham Flexner (1910, 19), wrote, "Indeed, the advertising methods of the commercially successful schools are amazing" and noted in a footnote that one school even offered a free trip to Europe to any student who attended for three years.

The Flexner report initiated a series of reforms that resulted in the regulated, modern form of medical education found in the US today (see chap. 1). Organized medicine developed rapidly during the twentieth century, establishing itself as objective, reliable, and trustworthy by severing its overt links with theater, showmanship, advertising, and profit. It largely succeeded, although echoes of theatrics and showmanship are still found in pharmaceutical pitches, nutritional supplement claims, and the like.[8] Evidence-based practices today rely on scientific research as the basis on which claims are made and protocols are developed. Extensive test trials are conducted before new drugs are released, and there are endless rules and regulations that govern recommended therapies. Medical knowledge is circulated through peer-reviewed journals, lectures, and public health campaigns, and the information is serious rather than entertaining in tone.

Today organized medicine lies fully within the realm of expert knowledge. As Michel Foucault argues in his book *Power/Knowledge* (1980), the ability to determine what counts as knowledge is closely related to power. Having established itself as an expert knowledge, modern medical knowledge is now also a form of power.

Ancient forms of the carnivalesque derided official truths, knowledge, and the power they represented. Bakhtin continuously emphasizes this point. He writes, for example, that the various figures who are uncrowned and abused in Rabelais's writings "are all subject to mockery and punishment as individual incarnations of the dying truth and authority of prevailing thought, law, and virtues" ([1968] 1984, 212). The medical carnivalesque derides the seriousness, authority, and power of contemporary expert medical knowledge by

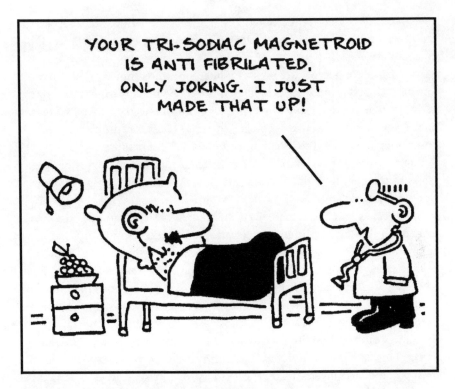

Figure 5.2. Cartoon poking fun of medical jargon.

reanimating medicine's older linkages to showmanship and profit, reframing it as spurious. Physicians make fun of themselves and the institutions in which they work, and they posit alternate knowledge formations that go directly against science. Through caricature, parody, satire, and play, expert knowledge is reframed as funny, nonsensical, or lacking practicality, while doctors themselves are portrayed as idle, greedy, or foolish.

Stereotypes and the Organization of Work

Caricatures of medical specialties offer particularly rich examples of how medical humor temporarily uncrowns official expertise. The medical world values intelligence, rationality, humility, ethics, and hard work, but in folklore certain specialties represent the opposite of those values: orthopedics represents a lack of intelligence; psychiatry represents insanity; surgery represents arrogance and greed; oncology represents a lack of ethics; anesthesiology represents idleness. The tag line for psychiatry in *Gomerpedia*, for example, is "Only consult between the hours of 11AM and 1PM," suggesting that psychiatry is easy because the doctors are only available for limited hours ("Psychiatry"). The entry for the American Academy of Orthopedic Surgeons states that in addition to "fixing, counting, throwing, juggling, or burying bones.... Ripping phone books in half is also a favorite pastime" ("American Academy"). This description alludes to the broad range of jokes about orthopedic surgeons as strong and somewhat dumb. The tag "Sudoku rules!" under anesthesiology refers to the common idea that anesthesiologists are idle and play games at work ("Anesthesiology").

Stereotypes emphasize perceived differences between groups. They arise in medicine because of differences in the organization of knowledge and work among specialties. All postgraduate medical training in the US (that is, training beyond medical school) is organized according to the specialty system. Each medical specialty deals with particular aspects of health and the body, and specialists are highly trained in that area. Even areas of medicine that have a broad knowledge base are specialties, such as family medicine. The training for specialties can overlap with each other (for example, a psychiatrist completes a year of internal medicine before entering a psychiatric residency), but for the most part modern physicians are trained according to specialties after medical school.

The result is that each specialty develops its own knowledge system and folk culture, with its own lingo, personality traits, and ways of communicating, including specific approaches understanding and managing health care. As observed by Anne Burson-Tolpin (1990, 82):

> Each specialty has its own peculiar subculture shaped by the perspectives of the specialty and by its practitioners' perceptions of the relative merits of other specialties. Surgery, for instance, takes an aggressively intervention-ist stance, sometimes, as those in the medical specialties would say, to the point of being "knife happy." Its subculture reflects this orientation through tongue-in-cheek sayings such as "First the incision, then the decision" or "Never let the skin get between you and the diagnosis." Surgery is a predomi-nantly male specialty, and its macho reputation likewise reflects this. Internal medicine, on the other hand, claims to be a more intellectually rigorous specialty, one whose practitioners usually prefer conservative management with drug and other therapies to surgical intervention. Its practitioners are reputed to be among the most "obsessive-compulsive" in medicine.

It is the differences in approaching, diagnosing, and managing health care that is the basis of folklore about medical knowledge, differences that are exemplified in the following saying:

> The surgeon knows everything and does everything
> The internist knows everything and does nothing
> And the psychiatrist knows nothing and does nothing. (Anonymous, interview, April 10, 2012)

Stereotypes about specialties arise in medical school. Howard S. Becker and colleagues (1961, 408–14) discuss such stereotypes as they existed in the mid-twentieth century, which included ideas about general surgery, internal medicine, pediatrics, and dermatology. These stereotypes still hold sway today. Students choose a specialty as they apply for residency spots (although students may apply for spots in more than one specialty), and they do so with only a little experience in that specialty during their M3 and M4 rotations. Choosing a specialty is a source of anxiety for medical students and as shorthand summaries of "information," stereotypes can be useful. When I asked students about stereotypes of specialties, I received similar answers. The ROAD specialties, for example, stood for radiology, ophthalmology, anesthesiology, and dermatology. When I asked what "ROAD" meant, one medical student stated, "Well-paying, low hours. It's like the road to riches, you know? The easy road, the road to riches" (anonymous, interview, March 22, 2012).

The stereotypes elicited were largely unflattering: pediatrics, for example, was for people who liked children but were not particularly smart, while surgery was for people who were "type A" personalities and liked to cut. Pathology was for "nerds" who lacked people skills because they have little or no patient contact. When I asked an M1 about pathology, for example, she replied: "[It's for] people who lack people skills, it's like 'Oh, you'd make a good pathologist.'" She later added, "It's kind of an insult when like someone says that you should be a pathologist, because that implies you don't have people skills" (anonymous, interview, March 21, 2012). Another student added, "Anesthesiologists and pathologists like their patients dead or asleep" (anonymous, interview, March 21, 2012).

Dermatology ("derm" for short), was a very competitive specialty at the time I conducted interviews in 2012. When I asked one medical student, "What about derm?" she replied, "[Derm] I would associate with people who want to make a lot of money without doing anything too hard" (anonymous, interview, March 21, 2012). Another said: "Derm, well, you have to be really smart to get into it, so there's that; but there's also the good lifestyle implications, and it seems like dermatologists are always very put together" (anonymous, interview, March 22, 2012). A few other students confirmed the idea that dermatologists "look good." In other words, dermatologists work with skin, and so one stereotype is that they are good-looking.

Psychiatry unsurprisingly was characterized as consisting of crazy people. I talked to an M4 who had just been accepted into a psychiatry residency. He was quite aware of the stereotype, noting that "you tell them [people] you're going into psychiatry and they're like 'What are you, nuts? Everybody that goes into psychiatry is insane,' you know? . . . I don't completely disagree [with the stereotype]. I think a lot of people that go into psychiatry do go into it because they're curious about their own problems . . . but there are a lot of weird people (myself included I guess) that go into psychiatry" (anonymous, interview, April 10, 2012). One medical student noted, "There's a stereotype that psychiatrists are like not—like, they're kind of weird" (anonymous, interview, March 21, 2012).

Stereotypes can provide the basis for wit. Like humor about patients, this wit does not target specific individuals but rather revolves around character types, with each specialty representing an idea or cluster of ideas (Cashman 2006). The M4 above, for example, provided several psychiatry jokes. "Like, somebody will say: Q: What's the difference between a psych patient and a psychiatrist? A: The psychiatrist has a key to the ward" (anonymous, interview, April 10, 2012). When I asked Dr. Mary Gibbs, a practicing psychiatrist in Salt Lake City, if she knew any psychiatry jokes she told me the following:

Q: How many psychiatrists does it take to change a light bulb?
A: Depends if the lightbulb wants to change. (Interview, September 7, 2019)

This example plays on the idea of what psychiatrists do, which is help patients change themselves.

There are humorous flowcharts based on stereotypes that "help" medical students decide, vis-à-vis a series of questions, for which specialty the student might be suited. One flowchart begins with the question: "What's the problem?" with the choice of answers being "I like everything" (in which case, one is directed to family medicine) or "I like nothing," which is then followed by a series of questions regarding grades, whether or not one likes to cut, whether one is a people person, and how much of nerd one might be. Huge nerds and those who dislike people are directed to pathology and neurology. Those who answer "Huh?" to a question about attention deficit hyperactivity disorder are directed into emergency medicine (described by one student as "kind of plug and chug . . . they just live on adrenaline" [anonymous, interview, March 22, 2012]). (As an aside, ER physician Dr. Elonen said that before she decided to do ER, an attending physician told her: "I don't know what field you're going to go into, but you are an adrenaline junkie" [Interview, June 19, 2020]). Those who answer that sleep is "for the weak" and "no" to the absurdist question "Do people say 'meow' when they see you?" are guided to general surgery. (Those who answer "go to hell" to this question are directed to ob-gyn.) Those who "like people" but are "unwilling to touch them" are directed into psychiatry (fig. 5.3).

There are variations of the specialty flowchart. One popular version starts with the question: "Crazy? Or not crazy?" In another version, the initial question asks whether or not the reader is a "people person" and from there one chooses whether or not one minds being vomited on, positive or negative responses to rashes and feet (a "yes" moves one into dermatology), and whether or not one is secretly a vampire (radiology, pathology). Those who don't secretly think they are vampire, don't sleep, and *can* see their reflection in a mirror become surgeons (fig. 5.4). Vampirism is associated with a number of specialties, including surgeons, anesthesiologists, radiology, and pathology. The association seems largely based on lack of sleep, a preference for working in dark rooms, and an interest in bodily fluids. Such flowcharts undermine the seriousness of medical expertise and decision-making by suggesting it is based on unrelated, nonsensical assortments of preferences.

The organization of medical work means that physicians who complete residencies and fellowships have highly detailed, technical, and specialized knowledge. But highly specialized physicians are also less knowledgeable about areas in which they have not trained. Orthopedics, for example, defers heart issues to cardiologists, while cardiologists only treat the heart. These knowledge boundaries can leave doctors with the impression that doctors outside their specialty don't know information they consider essential. This is why hospitals deliver patient care in teams. A patient who is admitted to the hospital for chronic obstructive pulmonary disease, for example, but who also has heart issues might have a pulmonologist as their attending physician (the person ultimately responsible for the patient's care), but that attending might call a number of "consults" (advice) for help with issues outside of pulmonology's areas of expertise. Such situations generate a robust body of esoteric-exoteric folklore based on presumptions by one group about themselves and others (and vice versa) that contributes to intergroup dynamics (Jansen 1959).

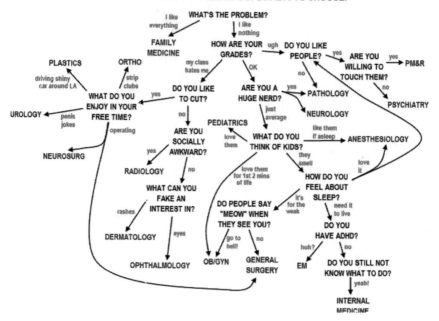

Figure 5.3. Flowchart for choosing a medical specialty.

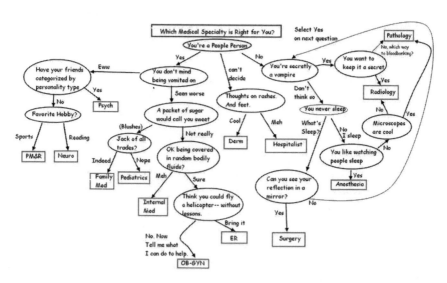

Figure 5.4. Variation of flowchart for choosing a medical specialty.

Targeting Expertise

Of all the specialties, orthopedic surgery seems the most maligned. Orthopedic surgeons (colloquially known as "orthopods") are targeted in jokes as being dumb. This is untrue: orthopedics is competitive and excellent board scores are required to secure a residency spot. But as the medical field values intelligence, it is unsurprising that some specialties are caricatured as lacking smarts. Noted joke scholar Christie Davies (2011, 20) writes that "stupidity" joke cycles targeting groups of people are common: "They are told about various groups and are told in many countries, indeed almost universally." He argues that groups who work with material objects often became the butt of stupidity jokes, and he uses orthopedic surgeons as an example, because bones are the most material aspect of the body: "Working with bones is seen as requiring mere physical strength and manual skill rather than a subtle understanding of medical processes" (23). The idea that orthopedists are unintelligent is found internationally: Davies provides a joke told to him by an Israeli physician in Hungary in 2007:

Q: What is a double-blind study?
A: Two orthopedic surgeons looking at an electrocardiogram. (23)

He concludes that "for the jokers, brainy surgeons work on brains and the bone-headed on bones" (24).

Orthopedic tools are quite "material" as well. Orthopedics is a surgical specialty, but alongside sophisticated computer equipment, miniature cameras, and delicate surgical instruments, standard orthopedic tool trays include large hammers, chisels, and various kinds of saws—the kinds of tools, an orthopedist told me, that one could buy at any Home Depot (also reported in Davies 2011, 24). It is said apocryphally that patients are put to sleep before the orthopedic tool tray is wheeled into the operating room because the tools used for surgery are so intimidating. (This is untrue; patients are anesthetized in the operating room and the tray is already there.) The type of tools used is one reason orthopedic surgeons are sometimes characterized (and characterize themselves) as "carpenters," that most material of all trades.

In addition to being caricatured as dumb, orthopedists are stereotyped as being strong. A certain amount of sheer strength is required for some kinds of orthopedic surgery, such as hip replacements and back surgery. Dislocating and removing a hip requires a lot of force. The requirement of strength is one reason sometimes given as to why there are fewer women in orthopedics, although other factors realistically play a more important role.[9] Orthopedics also is the specialty that covers sports-related injuries and sports medicine.

This fact, combined with ideas about "strength" and "lack of brains," means that orthopods are the jocks of the medical world. They suffer from the same image problems and stereotypes that jocks endure in society at large: the perception of a lack of intelligence and reliance on brute strength to get the job done.

These themes emerge in joke cycles. The joke below was told to me by a medical student:

> Q: Did you hear about the tragedy of the orthopedic department's library?
> A: There was a fire and it burned their one book. (Anonymous, interview, April 10, 2012)

The idea is that orthopedists don't read books, or are uninterested in learning, an orientation that goes directly against the core medical value of being educated and informed. A similar theme is found in the well-known "how do you hide a dollar from a doctor" joke cycle. The following question and response is given about orthopedists:

> Q: How do you hide a dollar from an orthopedist?
> A: Put it in a book.

The "hide-the-dollar" joke cycle is well known among doctors. Each example in the cycle targets a certain specialty, but the entire cycle targets all doctors as people who are money-hungry. Other examples from this joke cycle include the following:

> Q: How do you hide a dollar from a radiologist?
> A: Put it on a patient.

> Q: How do you hide a dollar from a general surgeon?
> A: Ahh, you *can't* hide a dollar from a general surgeon.

The radiologist joke refers to the fact that radiologists lack patient contact. The second example jibes surgeons as a specialty that is both extraordinarily skilled (that is, there is nothing they can't do, including find a dollar) and also especially greedy.

A similar set of responses are found in the joke cycle that asks how each kind of doctor saves the elevator door. The answer is the part of the body that specialty does not use.

> Q: How does an orthopedist save the elevator door?
> A: Uses their head.

Q: How does an internist save the elevator door?
A: Uses their hand.

Q: How does a surgeon save the elevator door?
A: Uses someone else. (Sheppard, interview, September 20, 2019)

The first joke amplifies the theme that orthopedists are dumb (they don't need the head), while the internist example plays on the fact that internists rarely do medical procedures and therefore don't need their hands. The surgery joke plays on the idea that surgeons are extraordinarily skillful and therefore "need" all of their body parts but also that they lack empathy and are willing to sacrifice someone else to save the door.

Online videos poke fun at orthopedics. One well-known video, uploaded in 2010 with 1.6 million views at the time this book was drafted, is an animated YouTube video called "orthopedics vs. anesthesia" (Tazobactar 2010). The video features a conversation between two unidentifiable animal forms, one of whom is an anesthesiologist and the other of whom is an orthopedist, specialties that work closely together during surgery and engage in friendly rivalry (see Dundes 1987, 101). The orthopedist asks the anesthesiologist to prepare a patient for surgery since the patient has a broken bone. The anesthesiologist then asks the orthopedist questions in order to determine whether or not the patient is suitable for anesthesia. In the exchange, it turns out that the orthopedist can't answer any questions about the patient: his only answer is to repeat the phrase: "There is a fracture. I need to fix it." The idea that orthopedists don't know anything medically about their patients is another stereotype: they are only interested in the specific limb on which they are operating. It is eventually revealed that the patient is dead. The anesthesiologist explains with exasperation: "She's not fit enough for a haircut, let alone an operation!" This fact doesn't matter to the orthopedist, however, who continues to insist: "There is a fracture. I need to fix it," an example of Henri Bergson's ([1900] 1937) idea that "rigidity" elicits laughter and comic response. The video also is funny to physicians because while anesthesiologists stereotype orthopods as lacking medical insight, orthopedic surgeons may consider anesthesiology annoying because they are picky about who might be fit for sedation, thus delaying surgery (the surgeon's goal). In the comments section, one contributor named 1fisiu posted the following (typos in original have been fixed): "Funny how well known this is among MDs even abroad. I'm doing internship in Sweden. (In Sweden internship year is separated from residency, which you apply for later.) On my ortho rotation at the ortho ER late in the evening, tired and all, after examining a patient I went to the doctor's lounge where my older colleagues doing ortho residency sit and said 'I have a fracture I need to fix it' and everyone fell in to laughter knowing exactly what it's all about."

The humor-generating rivalry between orthopedics and anesthesia also is found in published articles. The *BMJ* (formerly known as the *British Medical Journal*) published a tongue-in-cheek article in 2011 titled "Orthopaedic Surgeons: As Strong as an Ox and Almost Twice as Clever? Multicentre Prospective Comparative Study" that compared the IQs and "mean grip strength of the dominant hand" between orthopedists and anesthesiologists. Authored by orthopedists, the justification for the article according to the authors was that the "stereotypical image of the strong but stupid orthopaedic surgeon has not been subject to scientific scrutiny" (Subramanian et al. 2011, 1). Of course, the subtitle of the article, "Strong as an Ox and Almost Twice as Clever," is funny when one realizes the authors are orthopedists, as it still suggests that orthopedists aren't really smart—they are only "almost twice as clever" as an ox, although they are as strong as one. After outlining the study's methods, the authors note in the discussion section: "This study is the first of its kind to provide evidence for the perpetual banter between orthopaedic surgeons and anaesthetists. . . . with higher results for orthopaedic surgeons" (2). They conclude, "The stereotypical image of male orthopaedic surgeons as strong but stupid is unjustified in comparison with their male anaesthetist counterparts. The comedic repertoire of the average anaesthetist needs to be revised in the light of these data" (3).

The Amateur Transplants, a British singing group made up of anesthesiologists, wrote a popular song that pokes fun of orthopedics. The group wrote, performed, and recorded satirical songs about medical practice during the early 2000s. One of their most well-known songs, the "Drugs Song," is sung to the tune of Gilbert and Sullivan's 1879 "I am the very Model of a Modern Major-General," from the musical *The Pirates of Penzance*. Mathematician, performer, and satirist Tom Lehrer used the tune in 1959 to create "The Elements" song, in which he fired off at a very rapid pace the names of all 102 chemical elements that were known at the time: the song was something like a tongue twister or a challenge to see how quickly he could recite the periodic table. The Amateur Transplants likely used "The Elements" song as inspiration for their own version, in which they sing the names of over one hundred drugs in about one minute and forty-five seconds. The first two stanzas of the song are as follows:

There's aspirin, adrenaline, and also aminophylline
Amphetamine, adenosine, augmentin, and rifampicin

Amoxicillin, penicillin, heparin, and warfarin
And estrogen, progestogen, and canesten and chloroquine

There's bendroflumethiazide and also cyclophosphamide
And metoclopramide, acetazolamide, tropicamide
Loperamide, amiloride, and cyclizine and frusemide
And if you're up the duff then you'd best avoid thalidomide

The glory and cleverness of the song is the singer's ability to roll the names of difficult-to-pronounce drugs off the tongue. The alliteration and assonance of the vowels and consonants that make up the drug names are pleasing, and they fit neatly within the meter of the well-known tune. The last lines, however, provide the zinger. The song concludes:

You must remember all these drugs
the names of which you've learned from me [dramatic pause]
Or fuck it all and get a job in orthopedic surgery! (Take Aurally 2017)

This last line underlies the idea that if one does not have the ability to memorize all of the drug names, one can still go into orthopedic surgery, since knowing and understanding complex drugs is unnecessary.

Folklore targets other specialties as well. The main stereotype associated with psychiatry is that it attracts crazy people; it also is stereotyped as lacking medical expertise. When I asked Dr. Gibbs what the stereotypes were regarding psychiatry, she responded: "About psychiatry? That's a good question. I think one of the stereotypes is that we don't know how to do medicine. So, like if someone has a medical emergency, we don't handle it—we have 'real doctors' (if you will) take care of it, which isn't the case. But that's a stereotype." She added, "We handle all sorts of medical emergencies here, and we know how to handle it, and we handle it well, actually. And we have ongoing training—because it's not something we deal with every, single day like some specialties (like ER), you know? So, we do just have ongoing training, so we're ready to go when it does happen. And I would even say because of that, we might be even better at it, because we get the specialized training. But that's another issue" (interview, September 7, 2019).

The idea that psychiatrists aren't "real doctors" is exemplified in the following lines from a YouTube video produced by students at the University of Chicago Pritzker School of Medicine and posted on May 29, 2014. The song is sung to the popular Disney tune "Let It Go" from the movie *Frozen*.

The fourth code light in the MICU tonight
Not a fellow to be seen

This patient's in isolation
And his sputum's kind of green
His pulse is bounding like
There's something wrong inside
Couldn't name it though
Heaven knows I've tried

Don't let them in
Don't let them see
How I look up this stuff on WebMD
It's time to round my panic grows
Oh God this blows

I don't know, I don't know
Can't hold it back any more
I don't know, I don't know
Get me up and off this floor
I don't care what they're going to say
Let the bad grades come

I wanna do psychiatry anyway. (Beannie Meadow 2014)

The last line here suggests that bad grades (due presumably to lack of ability) really don't matter if one plans on doing psychiatry.

Anesthesia is another targeted specialty. A common idea about anesthesiologists is that they are lazy and/or lack professionalism, as in the following joke:

Q: What do you call an anesthesiologist in a suit?
A: Defendant.

In this question-and-answer joke, anesthesiologists are depicted as lacking in professionalism on two levels. First, it suggests they lack professionalism in terms of attire—that is, they rarely wear suits. Most doctors don't actually wear suits, but many wear ties. Anesthesiologists, however, apparently may come to work in jeans, and so they can give other physicians the impression that they dress too casually. The joke also suggests anesthesiologists lack competence because they are the subject of lawsuits—hence, the wordplay on "suit"—that is, the only time they are appropriately attired (in suits) is when they appear in court, in a (law)suit.

The notion that anesthesiologists are "slackers" stems from the organization of their work. The ability to work hard and put in long hours, frequently without proper sleep, is a core value in the medical profession. All doctors claim that they work hard. But perceptions of what constitutes hard work and which specialties "have it rougher" permeate medical culture, as a sort of macho one-upmanship that occurs. Anesthesiologists believe that they work as hard as anyone else, but perceptions among doctors who work with them may differ. For example, anesthesiologists put the patient to "sleep" (paralysis) before surgery, but once surgery begins their job is to maintain the patient's state of paralysis, which is done through auditory and visual monitoring of screens. The anesthesiologist may even occasionally leave the room during surgery to check on other patients, as Dr. York did when I shadowed him at the University of Utah OR in 2016. When I asked another anesthesiologist, Dr. Ashka Lawton, about the stereotypes of anesthesiologists, she replied: "Yeah. [Laughs.] We have a few. People think we just sit there and sleep. Or sit there and drink coffee. Or they think we play crossword puzzles or Sudoku, or some sort of game—but we're not; we're paying attention [laughs]." When I asked her why there was that perception, she replied:

> I mean, there are certainly cases where it probably looks like we're sitting there doing nothing. But you know, we're pretty vigilant, I would say, almost all of us here. Not only do you use your eyes, but you have to use your ears as well, to tune into the different noises. Because each, you know, vital—for instance a pulse-ox has a very distinctive sound. So, even if your back is turned and you're doing something else—whether you're putting in an IV, or readjusting something on the patient—you have to be able to pick up the nuances and the change in the tone that can happen if a patient, let's say, desaturates, or something happens. But I'm sure it looks like to other people that we're just sitting behind the drapes, doing nothing. Which you know, I can totally understand. (Interview, July 21, 2020)

Dr. Lawton's perception of other doctors' perceptions, what William Hugh Jansen (1959) called the esoteric-exoteric factor in folklore, was borne out in interviews with medical students. As one student told me when I asked her about anesthesia stereotypes, "They sleep all the time and play Sudoku on their iPhone and read a newspaper during the procedure and don't pay attention at all to what's happening. . . . They're the vampires because they're the ones who usually start IVs. . . . They get to take lunch breaks and bathroom breaks [because] pretty much a scrub tech or nurse can get someone to come give them a break" (anonymous, interview, April 10, 2012). Tellingly, this student was about to enter a general surgery residency. The anesthetists' mode of attending to the patient is perceived as a lack of attention and thus a lack of a work ethic by other doctors.

To counter this stereotype and illustrate that anesthetists actually "do something" the Amateur Transplants (themselves anesthesiologists) wrote a song called "The Anesthetists Hymn," sung to the tune of Bonnie Tyler's "Total Eclipse of the Heart." Of course, what anesthetists "do" in the song turns out mostly to be changing the lights, the TV, and the radio. It is a nice example of a specialty laughing at itself.

> Everybody wonders what anesthetists do
> While the patient is asleep
> Everybody wonders what we do for three hours
> While that machine goes beep
> Everybody reckons we drink coffee and we gossip
> And we're generally subversive
> Everybody reckons we do crosswords and Sudoku
> And we chat up all the nurses
>
> But do you really think that's all we do?
> Well let me tell you now it isn't true
> 'Cause we sometimes check the screen
> And every now and then we write stuff
> And if we have to intervene
> We inject a bit of white stuff
> And we often do alter the lights
> or the height of the bed
> Or fiddle with the radio, change the CD
> We even check the patient occasionally
> And if they move we'll turn up to vapor
> And then we go back to reading the paper
> 'Cause when the patient's asleep
> We just sit and listen to the beep
> We just sit and listen to the beep
>
> Once upon a time I took pride in my job
> But now I think it's time to depart
> 'Cause I just sit here every day and listen to blips of the heart . . . (Dr. Mefisto 2016)

The perceived lack of a work ethic is likely the underlying reason why the trope "blame anesthesia" exists throughout medicine. Anesthesia is scapegoated as always at fault (in jest) by both surgery and medicine and "blame anesthesia" is a unifying, rallying cry across both of those departments. Dr. Lawton stated:

AL: The surgeons are always making fun of us, so we always make fun of them [laughs].

LG: There's like a rivalry there, isn't there?

AL: Yeah—it's a friendly rivalry, I would say [laughs].

LG: Can you talk a little bit about that?

AL: Oh, I mean—everyone always blames anesthesia for everything (jokingly). (Interview, July 21, 2020)

When I asked Dr. Lawton why "blame anesthesia" was funny, she said that somebody always has to be blamed for something and it was easy to "blame anesthesia" because anesthesiologists work individually rather than on teams and so are easy targets. Part of this scapegoating also likely exists because of the power dynamics and rivalry between anesthesia and surgery: as noted previously, it is the anesthesiologist who decides whether surgery will occur. The anesthesiologist evaluates whether a patient is fit for surgery, and if the anesthesiologist determines the patient is too sick, the surgery will not proceed. From a surgical point of view, it is therefore easy to "blame anesthesia."

The hashtag #blameanesthesia in fact exists on both Twitter and Instagram, where one can find a plethora of medical memes and jokes that blame something on anesthesia. "Blame Anesthesia" has its own Facebook group, and there are a number of *GomerBlog* headlines that blame anesthesia, including, "CMS Creates New 'Blame Anesthesia' ICD-10 Codes" and "Anesthesia Goes on the Offensive and Blames Everybody Else" (Dr. 99 "Anesthesia"; "Breaking: CMS Creates"). The hashtag #blameanesthesia was amplified in digital media when Dr. Jerome Adams became the twentieth United States Surgeon General in 2017 and the first anesthesiologist to hold the position. During the 2020 pandemic, he recommended that all elective surgeries be canceled or postponed to stop the spread of COVID-19. This led to a meme that displayed his portrait and contained the lines, "First anesthesiologist Surgeon General / cancels all elective surgeries" (fig. 5.5), and it is funny to physicians because it references the stereotype that anesthesia too easily cancels surgeries. Adam's nomination also led to the *GomerBlog* headline, "Anesthesiologist Sworn in as Surgeon General, Immediately Goes on Break" (Dr. Glaucomflecken, n.d.).

Another specialty targeted in medical humor, although much less often, is oncology. Humor about oncologists is not as prevalent as humor about other specialties, presumably because oncologists deal with cancer, a deadly serious topic. The medical students I interviewed did not hold stereotypes about oncology, and jokes about oncology are harsher than jokes about other specialties. This is because while orthopedists represent stupidity and anesthesiologists

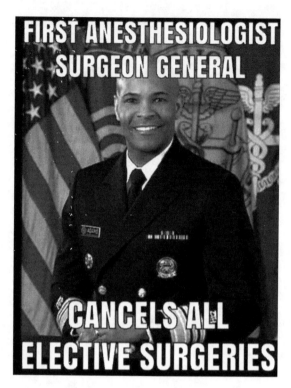

Figure 5.5. Meme amplifying "#blameanesthesia" when Dr. Adams became the first anesthesiologist to hold the position of US surgeon general.

represent idleness, oncologists appear to represent a lack of ethics, and ethics is probably the most fundamental of all medical values.

It is important to emphasize that the stereotypes represented in jokes are not true. As Alan Dundes (1987, 103) observed, stereotypes portray "traditional ideas about reality, not reality itself." Oncologists face difficult ethical decisions every day. They treat cancer by administering protocols that have severe side effects, and the death rate of cancer patients is high compared to other specialties. Quality-of-life decisions and issues of suffering are crucial. Life and death decisions about treatment, how long to continue treatment, and when to stop treatment can be wrenching for both patient and physician, and oncologists are highly aware of the ethical implications. For those outside of oncology, however, oncology can seem like a field in which treatment is harsh and may seem futile. The harmful effects of treatment may seem worse than death itself: this, of course, is the central issue in medical ethics. The following joke illustrates this perspective:

Q: Why do they put nails in a coffin?
A: To keep the oncologists out.

The joke suggests that oncologists insist on treating patients even after they are dead. It speaks to sensitive issues of whether to continue treatment when there is no longer hope, particularly when the treatment can cause suffering for the patient.

Problematic ethics are not limited to oncologists. The follow-up to the above joke is:

Q: What makes an oncologist madder than nails in a coffin?
A: When the note inside says, "Gone to dialysis."

This joke targets nephrologists, the doctors who order dialysis. The underlying perception played on in the joke is that nephrologists are always willing to put patients on dialysis—even, as the joke states, after they are dead. Both the initial joke and its follow-up speak to deep ethical issues about proper care for the very sick and dying that permeate medicine.

In sum, the folklore associated with various specialties targets medical knowledge/power. Medical specialties represent the pinnacle of expert knowledge, but in humor this expertise is lampooned, made nonsensical, or presented as inept, foolish, silly, or unnecessary, paralleling themes about physicians and academic medicine from earlier ages. The difference, however, is that contemporary humor about physicians emerges among doctors themselves. Calling one's own competence or the competence of one's peers into question in jest depends on a deeply situated sense of security in one's own expertise and in the expertise of others. The medical carnivalesque ultimately reinforces the aristocratic status of normative medical culture by positing the opposite in a comical way.

Alternative Knowledge: Beliefs about Luck

Another way in which expert knowledge is undermined in hospital settings is through ideas about luck. The general public would be surprised to hear that ideas about good and bad luck exist among physicians, who are characterized (and characterize themselves) as modern rationalists. Yet just as athletes, attorneys, and other professional groups have ideas about good and bad luck, physicians have a body of "superstitions" about what does and doesn't work at work. These superstitions are part of the occupational folklore of doctors, known and used across a wide variety of specialties.

Consider, for example, a text message I received from a physician friend on Friday the thirteenth in 2019: "Superstition is high at my work today: 13 new admits on Friday 13th with a full moon." This text refers to a complex of beliefs that the number thirteen is unlucky; that Friday the thirteenth traditionally is an unlucky day; and that a full moon adversely affects people's mental states. In this example, both the high number of admissions ("admits" or "hits") to the hospital as well as the fact that there were thirteen admissions specifically is "proof" of the bad luck.

This example is one of many. *Superstition* is an old term that has negative connotations in folklore studies, suggesting a false belief or idea that ignorant, uneducated people believe in. Superstitions supposedly are not based in logic, reason, or fact (although folklorists occasionally have shown otherwise), and so the term calls its own validity into question (Mullen 2000). Within a Western scientific perspective, a superstition by definition is not "knowledge," which is why the term is not often used by scholars: it pathologizes the folklore example as being wrong and sets up the group using the superstition as "different" from the rationalist, scientific scholar (Mullen 2000). Many scholars instead use the more neutral term *belief* or *folk belief*, recognizing that belief permeates all aspects of life, and they examine systems of belief instead of individual decontextualized "superstitious" examples.

In this case however, the term *superstition* is appropriate for two reasons. First, it is used by physicians themselves, as illustrated in the previous example of the text message. Second, physicians use the term *superstition* exactly *because* it signifies an explanation that is not based in "rational" or "expert" knowledge; superstitions are "spurious" knowledge. Physicians seek scientific-rationalist explanations of the world. In this occupational context of use, physicians use superstitions to purposefully and playfully amplify an alternative, spurious understanding of what is going on. Their own expert knowledge is made irrelevant, while "irrational" and "superstitious" beliefs like good luck, bad luck, full moons, jinxes, and Friday the thirteenth are drawn on as explanations for human behavior.

The moon plays a prominent role in hospital folk belief. It is a common idea among doctors, nurses, and other hospital staff that hospitals are "crazier" during a full moon. The modifier *crazy* can refer to either the behavior of patients or work that is chaotic, difficult, or unpredictable. This idea is found throughout different parts of the hospital, including the wards, the ER, the ICU, and, of course, the psychiatric unit. The moon complex includes ideas that there are more admissions into the hospital during a full moon; that those admissions are more complicated; that patients are noncompliant; and that there is an increase in suicides and psychiatric disturbances. Documented examples can also be found in the Wayland D. Hand Collection of Superstition and Popular Belief located in the Fife Folklore archives at Utah State University, such as "Belief that psychiatric patients get worse during a full moon."[10]

The idea that the moon holds sway over health is common enough that there have been studies conducted on whether or not patient behavior is affected by a full moon; whether the ER is busier; whether admissions to the hospital increase; and whether the moon affects surgery outcomes (e.g., Schuld et al. 2001; McLay, Daylo, and Hammer 2006; Gupta et al. 2019).[11] Studies concluded there is no correlation, but these ideas continue to exist nonetheless. For example, a psychiatrist forwarded me the following text they received from another physician as an example of a chaotic work environment blamed on the moon: "Is it a full moon? SK [initials of a patient] reported to staff tonight that she is making a 'pros and cons' list for killing herself and JC [initials of a patient] was taken to the ER" (anonymous, text communication, September 8, 2015).

The notion that the moon sways human behavior is called "the lunar effect" and dates to ancient times. The word *lunatic* in English refers to a person that is insane, but the original meaning of *lunatic* referred to insanity that depended on the phases of the moon. Examples of entries under "full moon" in the aforementioned Wayland D. Hand collection include "Marriages consummated at the full moon are the happiest" as well as "Love is attained through magic, especially to the full moon." Examples of the moon in relation to death include "A full moon means someone will die" and "Old people of extreme age are said to die at new of full moon."[12]

These examples suggest that moon's traditional domain is love, magic, and death. Love is a matter of human relationships, and magic traditionally is used to control forces beyond normal human capacities. The hospital is by nature a chaotic place where the world is out of order and events happen unexpectedly. People are admitted because their bodies or minds are not functioning, and death, while never routine, is always a possibility. The moon, then, as an astronomical body that influences matters of love, death, and magic, is an entity that, in tradition, is entirely wrapped up in matters of general well-being. It is therefore not surprising to find references to the moon in hospitals rather than references to other astronomical bodies such as the sun or the stars.

Superstitions also manifest in ideas about white and black clouds. This complex arises during training, as the ideas have to do with overbearing workloads. A physician during their training can be labeled as a "white cloud" or a "black cloud," an example of folk ideas about character framed in terms of weather (Laudun 2023). The white cloud/black cloud framework draws directly from traditional weatherlore, which is that white clouds signal fair weather, clear sailing, and good luck, while black clouds indicate foul weather and rough waters. When applied to physicians, the idea is that some people generate their own weather systems. A doctor who is a "white cloud" generates metaphorically clear and sunny weather in the hospital, meaning that the day runs quietly and smoothly. There are not many admissions or difficult patients, and nobody dies. Work is good. Physician-generated weather systems also affect coworkers. It is always desirable to work with someone who is a white cloud because one's own workload is easier. A doctor who is a white cloud brings good luck to the work environment. A black cloud, however, is a physician who brings bad luck to work by generating bad, stormy weather. Everyone's workload increases when a black cloud doctor is working. Admissions are relentless, patients code and die, and the overall environment is chaotic. Physicians do not want to work with someone who is a "black cloud" because their own day will be difficult.

A "black cloud" is similar to a jinx. The *OED*'s definition of *jinx* as a noun is "a person or thing that brings bad luck or exercises evil influence."[13] According to the Hand archive, both objects and people can be jinxes. The majority of objects connected to jinxes in the Hand archive were work-related and had military connotations. These included boats, as in "Even blessing of fleet fails to bring good luck to some boats," and airplanes, "Every squadron had a jinx aircraft. This is a plane that seems to get into trouble on every mission. . . ." People were also identified as jinxes, particularly people associated with mining, the air force, or sports. "No man will go on a voyage if he knows there is a man on board recognized as unlucky, or as they term him, a jinker"; and, "There are some people who in regard to mining, are born under an evil sign or jinx"; and "Certain crew members, commanding officers, or element leaders are [*sic*] sometimes considered jinxed [air forces]."[14]

The archival examples suggest that jinxes exist in high-stakes environments. In medicine, it also is possible to jinx one's shift by saying, for example, "It's kind of slow (or quiet) around here!" as inevitably it will become a busy night. This idea is found in the UK as well. Dr. Adam Kay (2017, 160) writes, "Say the Q-word [quiet] to a doctor and you're all but performing an incantation, summoning the sickest patients in the world to your hospital." Like ideas about the number thirteen and influences of the moon, jinxing one's workload also has been studied "scientifically." According to the authors of a 2021 study, the study "refutes the central dogma of all of medicine, which suggests that saying the word 'quiet' increases the clinician's workload during the working day" (Singh, Ferro, and Fowell 2021).

The white cloud/black cloud complex is not applied to nurses or other hospital staff because it is related to the organization of physician work. Doctors work in teams to admit people to the hospital, and the admitting team must take any patient who qualifies. There is no maximum number of patients that might be admitted. Admissions take a long time and so a large number of admissions means a lot of work. Doctors also are responsible for their patients even when they are not at the hospital, so having a lot of admissions means additional work even after one goes home. During a quiet night with few admissions, doctors can catch up on work, research their patients' problems, or even sleep. In contrast, nurses work in shifts; have a maximum number of patients they may care for; and are not responsible for patients after they leave the hospital. A black cloud is less relevant to their immediate workload.

Another reason that nurses and other hospital staff are not labeled as black or white clouds is due to power differences. Physicians have more power and status than other hospital workers. Labeling someone with less power and status as a "black cloud" would be disrespectful, condescending, and certainly asking for trouble. If a doctor finds out she or he is working with a "black cloud," they may blasphemy the black cloud's mother to their face or curse the day the black cloud was born, but such disparagement and insulting behavior can only exist among peers. Finally, the designation is only given by others: one would never label oneself a black or white cloud.

What hope does a black cloud have? What recourse? Colleagues may curse the day a black cloud was born, but it is not one's fault. Black clouds are not blamed for their condition; others just don't want to work with them. How a black cloud responds to their unhappy situation is important. If a black cloud responds to their relentless workload by rising to the occasion with a positive attitude, does a good job of taking care of a difficult, heavy load of patients, and does not make things worse for his or her peers than it already is, then the black cloud earns respect. The black cloud has responded to their terrible condition in the best way possible, proving beyond doubt that they are a good—even excellent—doctor because they work hard. Other doctors will recognize the good job the black cloud has done in the face of ongoing calamity and the black cloud's reputation will be enhanced. The black cloud/white cloud belief complex, then, in addition to providing alternative explanations for unseemly workloads, reinforces institutional norms by providing an opportunity to prove one's worth to peers by, yet again, doing large amounts of work.

Notes

1. *Gomerpedia* is done by the same creators as *GomerBlog*. See http://gomerpedia.org/wiki/Main_Page.

2. I am grateful to my colleague Dr. Phebe Jensen, Professor of English at Utah State University for the gloss on this quotation.

3. *Oxford English Dictionary*, s.v. "mountebank," last revised March 2003, https://www.oed.com/dictionary/mountebank_n?tab=meaning_and_use #35762376.

4. *Oxford English Dictionary*, s.v. "charlatan," last modified July 2023, https://www.oed.com/dictionary/charlatan_n?tab=meaning_and_use#9608410.

5. *Commedia dell'arte* is a theatrical form that emerged during the early modern period in Italy and eventually spread to the rest of Europe. It became particularly popular and well developed in France, where it was known as *comédie-Italienne*. It was based on stock characters and known sketches or scenarios already familiar to audiences but that also contained a large degree of improvisation. Actors were itinerant and performed wherever they could.

6. A similar character exists in the Doctor in English mummer's plays as well as in an Italian Lenten skit called "Saw the Old Woman" ("Sega La Vecchia"). As in the Italian commedia dell'arte, these plays utilize stock characters and traditional, improvised sketches. In the British versions, the Doctor is drunk, interested in money, and speaks nonsense words. His cures, although nonsensical, revive a dead man (Rudlin 1994). In "Saw the Old Woman," the Doctor cures the old woman, who has been sawed in half, with "strange and absurd medicines" (Siporin 2022, 51). My thanks to Steve Siporin for this Italian example.

7. Other examples of Molière's plays that concern themselves with medical farce include *La Jalousie du Barbouillé* (1660), which contains a character who is "an undisguised French version of the *commedia dell'arte* Dottor Graziano," (Andrews 2005, 448) and whose analysis of the problem completely misses the mark, and *La Malade imaginaire* (1673), in which a clever maid named Toinette disguises herself as a doctor.

8. The establishment of organized medicine as an authoritative project has never been fully accomplished. The rise of antivaccination movements, particularly during COVID-19, is a recent example of its incomplete status.

9. Orthopedics remains the specialty with the fewest female residents. In 2018, women accounted for about 14 percent of orthopedic surgery residents (Williams 2018).

10. Wayland D. Hand Collection of Superstition and Popular Belief, Folk Collection 36, Fife Folklore Archives, Special Collections and Archives, Utah State University. This collection contains decontextualized superstitions and popular beliefs drawn from published sources and oral sources. The collection

contains over six hundred thousand entries, listed alphabetically; beliefs are listed on 3×5 cards and fill ten file-card cabinets.

11. The fact that there are published studies by medical personnel on whether or not these beliefs are accurate indicates they are taken with some degree of seriousness. However, many of these studies are written in a playful or joking tone, so my conclusion is that ultimately, there is a degree of ambivalence surrounding them.

12. Wayland D. Hand Collection of Superstition and Popular Belief, Folk Collection 36, Fife Folklore Archives, Special Collections and Archives, Utah State University.

13. *Oxford English Dictionary*, s.v. "jinx." Modified in July 2023 but not yet revised, https://www-oed-com.dist.lib.usu.edu/dictionary/jinx_n?tab=factsheet #40395138.

14. Wayland D. Hand Collection of Superstition and Popular Belief, Folk Collection 36, Fife Folklore Archives, Special Collections and Archives, Utah State University.

Conclusion

Suffering and the Carnivalesque

The healing dimensions of medicine have long been of interest to folklorists. Much of this work historically focused on so-called folk aspects, meaning that early scholars documented traditional cures, remedies, healing practices, and associated beliefs considered to be outside of or distinct from formal academic medicine. Folklorist Wayland D. Hand, for example, prolifically published on folk medicine and belief from the 1940s through the 1980s (Yoder 1972; Hand 1980). The original, massive Folk Medicine and Belief Archive located at UCLA (now available online as part of the Archive of Healing at www.archiveofheal-ing.com) houses a plethora of folk medical practices and beliefs about health, medicine, and healing.

Over time, folklorists moved their attention from folk remedies and folk beliefs to more holistic approaches, including a recognition that health care in general is embedded in systems of belief. Anthropologist Charles Briggs (2012) charts this history closely, observing that folk healing practices came to be understood more in relation with, rather than distinct from, organized medicine. Inspired by the pioneering efforts of folklorist David Hufford (e.g., 1998), who argued that academic medicine itself was not culture free, scholars today often focus on the patient's point of view in relation to modern health care systems and on intersections, overlaps, and conflicts between vernacular perspectives and practices and those associated with modern health care systems (O'Connor 1995; Brady 2001). Scholarship on lay narratives of disease and epidemics, including COVID-19, continues this important work (Goldstein 2004; Kitta 2012; Blank and Kitta 2015; Lee 2014; Briggs and Mantini-Briggs 2003).

This project takes an occupational approach to health, but it too answers the call for understanding the cultural dimensions of medicine. Medicine is the most intimately human of all professions, attendant to all aspects of the body and, in particular, the fundamental life processes of birth, sickness, aging, and death; it cannot be other than profoundly cultural. I have focused on physicians and the traditionalized, folkloric, often humorous ways that they talk to each other, illustrating concretely the strikingly close parallels between this backstage talk and ancient manifestations of the carnivalesque. This "medical carnivalesque" (Gabbert and Salud 2009), a comic and aesthetic mode, is an important and unrecognized cultural dimension of medicine (Gabbert 2020). The pervasiveness of suffering is a second unrecognized cultural dimension. Medical training, physician experiences, the institutional organization of work, work-related attitudes and values, the nature of medical responsibility, and the precise, often transgressive aspects of medical work causes suffering in physicians. This suffering, coupled with the suffering of patients and the mandate of medicine to relieve suffering, means that suffering infuses nearly every aspect of the profession. It provides the deep context for the medical carnivalesque.

A carnivalesque approach to this material, however, is not the only one available. Humor theories generally emphasize superiority theory, release theory, and incongruity theory, all of which are applicable. Superiority theory dates to the classic period but is often attributed to Hobbes. It posits that people laugh at and feel superior to objects of their amusement, and it tends to emphasize aggression since the humor evolves from ridicule, mockery, and abuse. Henri Bergson's ([1900] 1937) theory of laughter, for example, suggests that laughter is a corrective mechanism, meaning that it functions as a means of social control. People who transgress social norms or are overtly rigid in their behavior are laughable, and the purpose of laughter is to reintegrate the individual back into society. Yet as Sheila Lintott (2016, 348) argues, superiority theory only explains some instances of humor, namely, "a *certain sort* of comic amusement we may have to *a certain kind* of humor" (see also Carroll 2003). Superiority theory is particularly applicable to medical humor when the target is patients, and scholars examining such material observe that it functions to solidify in-group identity (Gordon 1983; Odean 1995; Fox et al. 2003). But based as it is in ridicule, mockery, and abuse, this applicability does not mean the humor is not also carnivalesque.

The same can be said for release theory, which stems from the work of Sigmund Freud and emphasizes psychic energy. This approach is psychological and functionalist. Freud ([1905] 2003) found the comic (as in the telling of a joke) to be a temporary release of inhibitions. The psychic energy normally expended on repression is saved in his view, resulting in a pleasure of economy as the unconscious is allowed expression. Release theory presumes that humor helps people cope, express hostility, and alleviate stress. It is a kind of psychological safety valve for letting off steam. This perspective parallels the way in which pre-Lenten Carnival has been theorized as a social safety valve for the masses to let off steam against elites. Release theory is commonly applied to humor in medicine, and the doctors themselves say that humor helps them deal with the stressors of work.

Incongruity theory, which dates to Kant, addresses how specific examples actually operate,[1] postulating that the humor hinges on some kind of mismatch, the juxtaposing of two elements that are incongruous. Philosopher of aesthetics Noël Carroll (2003, 347) describes it as a deviation from norms, "a problematization of sense. This can occur when concepts or rules are violated or transgressed." Mary Douglas (1968, 364), without invoking incongruity theory specifically, observes that jokes have a subversive effect on the dominant structure of ideas. Folklorist Elliot Oring expanded the idea of incongruity, theorizing that the incongruity needs to be understood as appropriate in some way. He writes, "This perspective claims that all humor depends on the perception of an incongruity that can nevertheless be seen as somehow appropriate" (2011, 213). Incongruity theory is entirely compatible with a carnivalesque perspective because one way carnival is transgressive is by juxtaposing conventional categories and images. Much of the commentary in gross anatomy lab can be subsumed under this approach.

I have emphasized a carnivalesque orientation here, however, because a carnivalesque perspective more precisely captures the nature of backstage medical folklore and offers a more holistic interpretation of these materials. Superiority theories, release theories, and incongruity theories are applicable, but they do not finger the experiential, philosophical, epistemological, and existential dimensions of doctoring in the same way. A carnivalesque orientation specifically fits the practice of medicine because it is profoundly concerned with the body in its various grotesque manifestations, in its interconnectedness with life and death, and in its relation to institutional knowledge/power. The discourses of science and medicine are exercised in teaching hospitals, and a broad carnivalesque orientation emerges in response. Ancient elements and expressions have been updated and revised but remain relevant.

It is easy to romanticize the carnivalesque and scholars have pointed out that Bakhtin himself did so. Terry Eagleton (2019a, 32), for example, writes of Bakhtin's "wide eyed idealism." Characterized as a mode of free expression without regard for hierarchies, a means to overcome fear, and as emancipation from official doctrines, it is comforting (and romantic) to think of carnival as liberating and easy to overlook the means by which it is achieved. Carnival

modes are not pretty or always "funny" in the conventional sense; they are profoundly ambivalent since they degrade, lampoon, mock, disfigure, dethrone,
and slander. They can also be violent, because they tear down in order to build
up. Yet the utopian, transformative aspects of carnival remain important because it is there that ties between carnival and suffering become more apparent.
I conclude then with some speculation (rather than arguments) about how and
why suffering and the carnivalesque coexist and relationships between the two.

Suffering broaches issues of the spirit and is usually addressed through religion. The first truth of Buddhism, for example, is that "life is suffering," largely
caused by human attachment or revulsion. The Judeo-Christian theological
idea of theodicy directly addresses the question of suffering by asking: "If God
is good, why do people suffer?" But Christianity does not address suffering
through the comic (although apparently Zen Buddhism does). Christianity, in
fact, historically condemned mirth and laughter (Houck 2007; Joeckel 2008).
The reason is that in Western society, that which is important (such as suffering) is framed as "serious," while humor and laughter are framed as "nonserious," a term that often implies "unimportant." At various times throughout
history, mirth and laughter were considered sinful or implied a lack of control.

The Judeo-Christian tradition relieves suffering by connecting individual
suffering to the suffering of Christ. This move transforms the suffering into
"something else," such as a test, punishment, correction, or opportunity. In the
book of Job, a primary religious text on suffering, Job's suffering at the hands
of God is explained (and so transformed) as a test and opportunity for growth.
Personal transformation also can be an outcome of suffering—one becomes a
better human being, rearranges life priorities, or maintains a closer relationship
with God. Such transformation may be accomplished through the ritual genres,
which manifest an alternative reality that is serious and permanent: social and
cultural categories, interpretations, and understandings of the world are reinforced and authorized through the invocation of a sacred, transcendent power.

The play genres, under which different kinds of humor fall, also create
alternate realities, but the transformation is temporary. Participants act as if the
meanings presented in play were true, although participants also acknowledge
that what is presented is, in fact, not true (Bateson [1972] 2000). This paradox
is vital because the invocation of an alternate, nonserious reality allows for a
broad range of experimentation, since what is done in play "doesn't count"
and so serious aspects of cultural and social life may be toyed with. Forms of
humor, playful speech, and various joking behaviors are mechanisms for changing given meanings by temporarily overturning, reframing, and challenging
the given interpretation of situations. Such devices reveal the ambiguity of

language and provide alternate, comic viewpoints, providing a shift of insight into what is going on. This is why Douglas (1968, 365, 366) comments that a joke "changes the balance of power" and that "its form consists of a victorious tilting of uncontrol over control, it is an image of the leveling of hierarchy, the triumph of intimacy over formality, of unofficial values over official ones."

The creation of alternate realities, whether accomplished through ritual or play, ultimately offers glimpses of transcendence. Sociologist and theologian Peter L. Berger (1997) defines *transcendence* in religious contexts as indexing another world that is redemptive, that has been made whole, or in which the mysteries of the human condition are abolished. Religious transcendence is by definition a world without suffering because "the promise of redemption . . . is always of a world without pain" (195). Comic modes such as the medical carnivalesque similarly index a "world beyond" because pain and suffering do not exist in the comic mode. Following Aristotle, Berger points out that "the comic presents a world without pain. . . . It is, above all, an abstraction from the tragic dimension of human experience" (194). He writes: "Generally, any comedy turns into tragedy as soon as real suffering, real pain is allowed to enter it" (195).

The medical carnivalesque reflects the realities of medicine because it is based on the body, but it creates a comic alternate reality in which suffering does not exist, reframing difficult, uncomfortable, or impossible situations to create new meanings. It reveals the difficult medical world as silly, banal, irreverent, and absurd. It transforms dominant frameworks from ones that assign sadness, grief, and failure to patient pain, illness, and death into ones that are irreverent; from frameworks that construct physicians as heroic and all-knowing to ones that construct them as quacks; from ones that emphasize the sacredness of the patient body to ones that frame it as a comic monster; and from frameworks that emphasize the work of doctors as gods to ones that posit them as fools who traffic in urine and feces for love of money. The meanings generated are silly or absurd, but they are not meaningless. The medical carnivalesque transforms the seriousness, pain, and suffering of the medical workaday world into a ludic one and so intimates transcendence.

This transformation is partially explained by release theory, which offers functional and psychological explanations. Release theory states that humor expresses forbidden anxiety, hostility, and other repressed or forbidden emotions and attitudes and so offers relief from the situation at hand. This is certainly true: by transforming work situations into a comic mode, physicians temporarily rid their workaday world of pain and create worlds in which suffering no longer exists. But the medical carnivalesque also offers glimpses of transcendence and so is a spiritual way out. Grounded as it is in the Cartesian mind/body split, medicine does not directly address the spiritual aspects of suffering but the pervasive, ludic, and carnivalesque mode indirectly does. Mary Douglas (1968, 374) comes to similar conclusions regarding jokes: "By revealing the arbitrary, provisional nature of the very categories of thought, by lifting their pressure for a moment and suggesting other ways of structuring reality, the joke rite . . . hints at unfathomable mysteries." Carnival, in its profound ambivalence and with its capacity for renewal and change, is a powerful weapon in medical contexts.

The broader implications of these connections additionally suggest that ancient forms of the carnivalesque are also concerned with suffering. Bakhtin insisted that carnival transformed existential terror, such as the terror of the grave and of natural forces. He repeatedly writes that carnivalesque laughter transformed terror into a "gay monster," meaning something terrifying (a monster) had been transformed into something comic, a merry thing to be laughed at that was no longer threatening. My research reveals that at least in medicine, the carnivalesque is related to real pain, death, and suffering, experiences that religion traditionally identifies as arenas for transcendence and so are also subjects that are connected to the sacred. Future explorations of other manifestations of the carnivalesque need to account for the role of suffering as well as its transcendent, potentially sacred nature.

Organizing Medicine

I conclude with a plea for society to take better care of its doctors, care that would necessarily involve systematic and institutional change. The global spread of COVID-19, which occurred as this book was being drafted, laid bare many core problems. Hospitals and staff were strained, in many cases beyond the breaking point. Physicians in different places and at different times throughout the nation implemented crisis standards of care, meaning that they had to make painful, morally injurious decisions about who would and would not receive resources. Doctors who did not work in hospitals could not get care for their patients, some of whom desperately needed it and were sent home to die. Caregivers were not just stressed or burned out; they worked—and continue to work—in an ongoing state of horror, pain, shame, exhaustion, anger, and frustration. COVID-19 is an extreme example, but the dynamics of the global pandemic only exacerbated and made obvious many of the already-existing issues in the nation's health care system.

There has been increasing acknowledgment in recent years that the nation's physicians are at serious risk. In the conclusion to his book *The Secret Language of Doctors*, Dr. Brian Goldman argues that medical slang is rooted in problems inherent to the institution and practice of medicine, which he states can produce "misery" in its doctors (39). Similarly, Dr. Abraham Verghese, reflecting on his physician friend's suicide in the book *The Tennis Partner*, observes a "terrible collusion to cover up pain, to cover up depression" in the medical field but also states that it is not the fault of individual physicians but rather the system that has been created (1998, 341). To date, however, the majority of strategies for improvement have focused on individual responsibility rather than systematic change. Strategies include encouraging physicians to participate in mindfulness activities like yoga and meditation, to undergo resiliency training, and to seek counseling or therapy. Such activities can be beneficial, but these solutions place responsibility for solving the problem on the physician. The reality is that most physicians are quite resilient, and practically speaking, the organization of work does not allow for wellness; that is part of the problem. Further, as Dr. Pamela Wible has argued, locating solutions for the ills of the nation's health care system in individual activities can be a subtle form of victim blaming: when physicians cannot make time for themselves due to work obligations, they can easily be faulted for their own failures (Symon 2018).

What is needed is institutional change, beginning with a recognition that suffering is part and parcel of doctoring. Only then can systemic approaches focus on changing how institutional work and training operate to lessen that suffering. Such change would entail a rehaul of the nation's entire health care system, including how medical students are educated, the organization of residencies, the influence of health insurance companies, and the ways in which hospitals typically are run. A robust health care system should ensure that its caregivers are healthy, physically, mentally, and spiritually. To accomplish this, doctors would likely need to unionize, an unlikely event. It also would entail a change in the culture of doctoring itself, from one in which extreme self-sacrifice and self-denial are valued as heroic to one in which a physician's strength is defined by the ability to recognize and address their own needs. It is a daunting task but not impossible. In the meantime, physicians find the medical carnivalesque a useful, alternative means of grappling with the challenges of medicine.

Notes

1. Other approaches deal with joke mechanics, such as the general theory of verbal humor (Attardo 2011).

REFERENCES

AAMC. 2018. "Report: An Updated Look at the Economic Diversity of U.S. Medical Students." *Analysis in Brief* 18 (5). https://www.aamc.org/data-reports /analysis-brief/report/updated-look-economic-diversity-us-medical -students.

————. 2022a. "2022 FACTS: Applicants and Matriculants Data." Table A-9, A-7.2. Accessed July 5, 2023. https://www.aamc.org/data-reports/students -residents/data/2022-facts-applicants-and-matriculants-data.

————. 2022b. "2022 FACTS: Enrollment, Graduates, and MD-PhD Data." Table B-4. Accessed July 5, 2023. https://www.aamc.org/data-reports/students -residents/data/2022-facts-enrollment-graduates-and-md-phd-data.

————. 2023. "Report: Tuition and Student Fees Reports." March. Accessed July 5, 2023. https://www.aamc.org/data/tuitionandstudentfees/.

Aasland, Olaf G., Erlend Hem, Tor Haldorsen, and Øivind Ekeberg. 2011. "Mortality among Norwegian Doctors 1960–2000." *BMC Public Health* 11:173. https://doi.org/10.1186/1471-2458-11-173.

American Foundation for Suicide Prevention. 2008. *Struggling in Silence: Physician Depression and Suicide.* 54 minutes, featured on PBS. DVD.

Andrews, Richard. 2005. "Molière, Commedia dell'Arte, and the Question of Influence in Early Modern European Theatre." *Modern Language Review* 100 (2): 444–63.

Anspach, Renee R. 1988. "Notes on the Sociology of Medical Discourse: The Language of Case Presentation." *Journal of Health and Social Behavior* 29 (4): 357–75.

Apte, Mahadev L. 1985. *Humor and Laughter: An Anthropological Approach.* Ithaca, NY: Cornell University Press.

Ariès, Philippe. 1975. "The Reversal of Death." In *Death in America*, edited by David E. Stannard, 134–58. Philadelphia: University of Pennsylvania Press.

———. 1981. *The Hour of Our Death*. Translated by Helen Weaver. New York: Knopf.

Attardo, Salvatore, ed. 2011. "The General Theory of Humor, Twenty Years After." Special issue, *Humor: International Journal of Humor Research* 24 (2): 123–262.

Bailey, Eleanor, Jo Robinson, and Patrick McGorry. 2018. "Depression and Suicide among Medical Practitioners in Australia." *Internal Medicine Journal* 48 (3): 254–58. https://doi.org/10.1111/imj.13717.

Bailey, Melissa. 2020. "Beyond Burnout: Doctors Decry 'Moral Injury' of Health Care System." *US News & World Report*, February 4, 2020. https://www.usnews.com/news/healthiest-communities/articles/2020-02-04/beyond-burnout-doctors-decry-moral-injury-from-health-care-financial-pressures.

Bakhtin, Mikhail. (1968) 1984. *Rabelais and His World*. Translated by Hélène Iswolsky. Bloomington: Indiana University Press.

Barkley, Dorothy. 1927. "Hospital Talk." *American Speech* 2 (7): 312–14. https://doi.org/10.2307/452893.

Bateson, Gregory. (1972) 2000. "A Theory of Play and Fantasy." In *Steps to an Ecology of the Mind*, 314–28. Chicago: University of Chicago Press.

Beannie Meadow (@bluebean10). 2014. "I Don't Know—Med School Parody of 'Let It Go' from Frozen (University of Chicago Pritzker SOM)." May 29, 2014. YouTube video, 3:45. https://www.youtube.com/watch?v=EtAG3e3JLNI.

Becker, Howard S. 1993. "How I Learned What a Crock Was." *Journal of Contemporary Ethnography* 22 (1): 28–35.

Becker, Howard S., Blanche Geer, Everett C. Hughes, and Anselm L. Strauss. 1961. *Boys in White: Student Culture in Medical School*. Chicago: University of Chicago Press.

Bendjelid, K. 2015. "The 'Hero Syndrome': A Human Condition of the ICU?" *Acta Anaesthesiologica Scandinavica* 59 (5): 677–78. https://doi.org/10.1111/aas.12514.

Bengtsson, Staffan, and Pia H. Bülow. 2016. "The Myth of the Total Institution: Written Narratives of Patients' Views of Sanatorium Care 1908–1959." *Social Science & Medicine* 153:54–61. https://doi.org/10.1016/j.socscimed.2016.02.005.

Berger, J. T., J. Coulehan, and C. Belling. 2004. "Humor in the Physician-Patient Encounter." *Archives of Internal Medicine* 164 (8): 825–30. https://doi.org/10.1001/archinte.164.8.825.

Berger, Peter L. 1997. *Redeeming Laughter: The Comic Dimension of Human Experience*. New York: Walter de Gruyter.

Bergman, Stephen. 2019. "Basch Unbound—The House of God and Fiction as Resistance at 40." *JAMA* 322 (6): 486–87. https://doi.org/10.1001/jama.2019.9499.

Bergson, Henri. (1900) 1937. *Laughter: An Essay on the Meaning of the Comic.* Translated by Cloudesley Brereton and Fred Rothwell. New York: Macmillan.

Blank, Trevor J. 2013. *The Last Laugh: Folk Humor, Celebrity Culture, and Mass-Mediated Disasters in the Digital Age.* Madison: University of Wisconsin Press.

Blank, Trevor J., and Andrea Kitta. 2015. *Diagnosing Folklore: Perspectives on Disability, Health, and Trauma.* Jackson: University Press of Mississippi.

Block, Melissa. 2004a. "First-Year Med Students Enter the 'Gross' Lab." NPR's *All Things Considered,* September 17, 2004. https://www.npr.org/2004 /09/17/3924247/first-year-med-students-enter-the-gross-lab.

———. 2004b. "Lessons from the Gross Anatomy Lab." NPR's *All Things Considered,* November 1, 2004. https://www.npr.org/2004/11/01/4136864 /lessons-from-the-gross-anatomy-lab.

Bracciolini, Poggio. 1879. *The Facetiae or Jocose Tales of Poggio.* Vol. 1. First translated into English with the Latin Text in Two Volumes. Paris: Isidore Liseux. http://hdl.handle.net/2027/uc1.b000949331.

Brady, Erika, ed. 2001. *Healing Logics: Culture and Medicine in Modern Health Belief Systems.* Logan: Utah State University Press.

Briggs, Charles L. 2012. "Toward a New Folkloristics of Health." *Journal of Folklore Research* 49 (3): 319–45. https://doi.org/10.2979/jfolkrese.49.3.319.

Briggs, Charles L., and Clara Mantini-Briggs. 2003. *Stories in the Time of Cholera: Racial Profiling during a Medical Nightmare.* Berkeley: University of California Press.

Brock, Alexander. 2008. "Humor, Jokes, and Irony versus Mocking, Gossip, and Black Humor." In *Handbook of Interpersonal Communication,* edited by Gerd Antos and Eija Ventola, 541–65. Berlin: De Gruyter. https://doi.org/10.1515 /9783110211399

Brock, D. Heyward. 1991. "The Doctor as Dramatic Hero." *Perspectives in Biology and Medicine* 34 (2): 279–95. https://doi.org/10.1353/pbm.1991.0018.

Brodie, Ian. 2014. *A Vulgar Art: A New Approach to Stand-Up Comedy.* Jackson: University Press of Mississippi.

Bronner, Simon. 1981. "The Paradox of Pride and Loathing, and Other Problems." *Western Folklore* 40 (1): 115–24.

———, ed. 2005. *Manly Traditions: The Folk Roots of American Masculinities.* Bloomington: Indiana University Press.

Brunk, Doug. 2015. "Physician Suicide: Common and Closeted." *Chest Physician* 10 (2): 20, 22.

Budd, Ken. 2020. "7 Ways to Reduce Medical School Debt." AAMC News, October 14, 2020. https://www.aamc.org/news-insights/7-ways-reduce -medical-school-debt.

Buehrer, David. 2017. "A World 'Funny as Shit': Black Humor and the New Naturalism in Harry Crews's *Feast of Snakes*." *Journal of the Georgia Philological*

Association 6:28–46. https://www.mga.edu/arts-letters/english/gpa/docs/jgpa -vol-6-2016-17.pdf.

Burson-Tolpin, Anne. 1989. "Fracturing the Language of Biomedicine: The Speech Play of U.S. Physicians." *Medical Anthropology Quarterly* 3 (3): 283–93. https://doi.org/10.1525/maq.1989.3.3.02a00070.

———. 1990. "'Fascinomas' and 'Horrendiomas': The Occupational Language, Humor, and Speech Play of American Physicians." PhD diss., University of Pennsylvania.

Caan, Woody. 2019. "GP Suicides: Lack of Support for Female Doctors." *BMJ* 365:l1908. https://doi.org/10.1136/bmj.l1908.

Campbell, Patrick. 2019. "Physician Suicide Remains a Misunderstood Problem." *HCPLive*, April 12, 2019. https://www.hcplive.com/view/physician-suicide -remains-a-misunderstood-problem.

Carroll, Noël. 2003. "Humour." In *The Oxford Handbook of Aesthetics*, edited by Jerrold Levinson, 344–365. Oxford: Oxford University Press.

Cashman, Ray. 2006. "Dying the Good Death: Wake and Funeral Customs in County Tyrone." *New Hibernia Review* 10 (2): 9–25.

Cassell, Eric J. (1991) 2004. *The Nature of Suffering and the Goals of Medicine.* 2nd ed. New York: Oxford University Press.

Center, Claudia, Miriam Davis, Thomas Detre, Daniel E Ford, Wendy Hansbrough, Herbert Hendin, John Laszlo, et al. 2003. "Confronting Depression and Suicide in Physicians: A Consensus Statement." *JAMA* 289 (23): 3161–66. doi: 10.1001/jama.289.23.3161.

Charon, Rita. 1986. "To Render the Lives of Patients." *Literature and Medicine* 5:58–74.

Christensen, Don. 1988. "Mirror, Mission, and Management: Reflections on Folklore and Culture in a Health Care Organization." In *Inside Organizations: Understanding the Human Dimension*, edited by Michael Owen Jones, Michael Dane Moore, and Richard Christopher Snyder, 49–61. Newbury Park, CA: Sage Publications.

Conrad, Susie. 2019. Recorded interview by Lisa Gabbert, December 8, 2019. Salt Lake City, UT.

Coombs, Robert H., Sangeeta Chopra, Debra R. Schenk, and Elaine Yutan. 1993. "Medical Slang and Its Functions." *Social Science & Medicine* 36 (8): 987–98. https://doi.org/10.1016/0277-9536(93)90116-L.

Corgain, Doug. 2019. Recorded interview by Lisa Gabbert, December 19, 2019. Salt Lake City, UT.

Curtis, J. Randall, and Mitchell M. Levy. 2014. "Our Responsibility for Training Physicians to Understand the Effect Patient Death Has on Them: The Role of the Intensivist." *Chest* 145 (5): 932–34. doi: 10.1378/chest.13-2600

Dans, Peter E. 2002. "The Use of Pejorative Terms to Describe Patients: 'Dirtball' Revisited." *Baylor University Medical Center Proceedings* 15 (1): 26–30.

Davies, Christie. 2011. *Jokes and Targets*. Bloomington: Indiana University Press.

Davis, Chelsea. 2020. "Sicko Doctors: Suffering and Sadism in 19th-Century America." *Public Domain Review*, July 1, 2020. https://publicdomainreview.org /essay/sicko-doctors.

Davis, Natalie. 1978. "Women on Top: Symbolic Sexual Inversion and Political Disorder in Early Modern Europe." In *The Reversible World: Symbolic Inversion in Art and Society*, edited by Barbara A. Babcock, 147–90. Ithaca, NY: Cornell University Press.

DeSole, Daniel E., Philip Singer, and Samuel Aronson. 1969. "Suicide and Role Strain among Physicians." *International Journal of Social Psychiatry* 15 (4): 294–301. https://doi.org/10.1177/002076406901500407.

dethorne. 2015. "The Diary of a Resurrectionist: The Value of Death." *UT Health San Antonio: The Libraries* (blog), April 30, 2015. http://library.uthscsa.edu /2015/04/the-diary-of-a-resurrectionist-the-value-of-death/.

DeZee, Kent J., Anthony R. Artino, D. Michael Elnicki, Paul A. Hemmer, and Steven J. During. 2012. "Medical Education in the United States of America." *Medical Teacher* 34 (7): 521–25.

Dholakia, S., P. J. Friend, and L. Maguire. 2016. "A Christmas Renaissance." *BMJ* 355:i6603. https://doi.org/10.1136/bmj.i6603.

Donnelly, William J. 1986. "Medical Language as Symptom: Doctor Talk in Teaching Hospitals." *Perspectives in Biology and Medicine* 30 (1): 81–94.

Doolittle, Benjamin. 2017. "ACGME Duty Hours Not the Only Big Change in Requirements." *NEJM Knowledge+* (blog), May 25, 2017. https:// knowledgeplus.nejm.org/blog/acgme-duty-hours-not-the-only-big-change-in -requirements/.

Douglas, Mary. (1966) 2003. *Purity and Danger: An Analysis of Concepts of Pollution and Taboo*. London: Routledge.

———. 1968. "The Social Control of Cognition: Some Factors in Joke Perception." *Man* 3 (3): 361–76.

Dowd, Maureen. 2011. "Decoding the God Complex." *New York Times*, September 27, 2011, sec. Opinion.

Dr. 99. n.d. "Anesthesia Goes on the Offensive & Blames Everybody Else." *GomerBlog*. Accessed July 10, 2023. https://gomerblog.com/2019/04/anesthesia -blames-everybody-else/.

———. n.d. "Breaking: CMS Creates New Blame Anesthesia ICD-10 Codes." *GomerBlog*. Accessed July 10, 2023. https://gomerblog.com/2018/06/blame -anesthesia-icd-10-codes/.

———. n.d. "Breaking News: THE PATIENT POOPED!!!" *GomerBlog*. Accessed June 14, 2020. https://gomerblog.com/2016/03/breaking-news-he -pooped/.

Dr. Glaucomflecken. n.d. "Anesthesiologist Sworn in as Surgeon General, Immediately Goes on Break." *GomerBlog*. Accessed July 10, 2023. https://gomerblog

.com/2017/09/anesthesiologist-sworn-surgeon-general-immediately-goes
-break.

Dr. Mefisto (@dr.mefisto7788). 2016. "AMATEUR TRANSPLANTS Anaesthetists Hymn LIVE." December 29, 2016. YouTube video, 1:49. https://www
.youtube.com/watch?v=g4fNaIurbo4.

Duchartre, Pierre Louis. 1966. *The Italian Comedy: The Improvisation, Scenarios,
Lives, Attributes, Portraits, and Masks of the Illustrious Characters of the Commedia dell'Arte.* Translated by Randolph T. Weaver. New York: Dover Publications.

Duncan, Chip, dir. 2018. *The First Patient.* Ro*Co Films. 1 hour, 20 minutes.
https://video.alexanderstreet.com/watch/the-first-patient.

Dundes, Alan. 1987. *Cracking Jokes: Studies of Sick Humor Cycles & Stereotypes.*
Berkeley, CA: Ten Speed Press.

Dundes, Alan, and Thomas Hauschild. 1983. "Auschwitz Jokes." *Western Folklore*
42 (4): 249–60. https://www.jstor.org/stable/1499500.

Dundes, Alan, and Carl R. Pagter. 1975. *Urban Folklore from the Paperwork Empire.* American Folklore Society: University of Texas Press.

Dundes, Lauren, Michael B. Streiff, and Alan Dundes. 1999. "'When You Hear
Hoofbeats, Think Horses, Not Zebras': A Folk Medical Diagnostic Proverb."
Proverbium: Yearbook of International Proverb Scholarship 16:95–103.

Duran, Alisa. 2019. "Breaking the Silence." *JAMA* 321 (4): 345–46. https://doi.org
/10.1001/jama.2018.22266.

Dutheil, Frédéric, Claire Aubert, Bruno Pereira, Michael Dambrun, Fares
Moustafa, Martial Mermillod, Julien S. Baker, et al. 2019. "Suicide among Phy-
sicians and Health-Care Workers: A Systematic Review and Meta-Analysis."
PLoS ONE 14 (12). https://doi.org/10.1371/journal.pone.0226361.

Eagleton, Terry. 2019a. *Humour.* New Haven, CT: Yale University Press.

———. 2019b. "The Politics of Humor: Whose Laugher, Which Comedy?" *Com-
monweal Magazine,* May 6, 2019. https://www.commonwealmagazine.org
/whose-laughter-which-comedy.

Ellison, Ed. 2017. "Doctors in Distress: How Do We Save the Lives of Those Who
Save Lives?" November 2017. TEDxNaperville. Accessed July 10, 2023. https://
www.ted.com/talks/dr_ed_ellison_doctors_in_distress_how_do_we_save
_the_lives_of_those_who_save_lives.

Elonen, Maija. 2020. Recorded interview by Lisa Gabbert, June 19, 2020. Salt
Lake City, UT.

Epstein, Ronald M., and Michael S. Krasner. 2013. "Physician Resilience: What
It Means, Why It Matters, and How to Promote It." *Academic Medicine* 88 (3):
301–3. https://doi.org/10.1097/ACM.0b013e318280cff0.

Falassi, Alessandro. 1987. "Festival: Definition and Morphology." In *Time Out of
Time: Essays on the Festival,* edited by Alessandro Falassi, 1–10. Albuquerque:
University of New Mexico Press.

Ferrari, Giovanna. 1987. "Public Anatomy Lessons and the Carnival: The Anatomy Theatre of Bologna." *Past & Present*, no. 117: 50–106. https://www.jstor.org/stable/650788.

Finkelstein, Peter, and Lawrence H. Mathers. 1990. "Post-Traumatic Stress among Medical Students in the Anatomy Dissection Laboratory." *Clinical Anatomy* 3 (3): 219–26. https://doi.org/10.1002/ca.980030308.

Flexner, Abraham. 1910. *Medical Education in the United States and Canada: A Report to the Carnegie Foundation for the Advancement of Teaching.* Carnegie Foundation Bulletin Number 4.

Foucault, Michel. 1973. *The Birth of the Clinic: An Archaeology of Medical Perception.* Translated by A. M. Sheridan Smith. New York: Vintage Books.

———. 1977. *Discipline and Punish: The Birth of the Prison.* Translated by Alan Sheridan. New York: Pantheon Books.

———. 1980. *Power/Knowledge: Selected Interviews and Other Writings, 1972–1977.* Edited by Colin Gordon. Translated by Colin Gordon, Leo Marshall, John Mepham, and Kate Soper. New York: Pantheon Books.

Fox, Adam T., Michael Fertleman, Pauline Cahill, and Roger D. Palmer. 2003. "Medical Slang in British Hospitals." *Ethics & Behavior* 13 (2): 173–89. https://doi.org/10.1207/S15327019EB1302_04.

Freud, Sigmund. (1905) 2003. *The Joke and Its Relation to the Unconscious.* Translated by Joyce Crick. New York: Penguin Classics.

Frye, Steven. 2019. Recorded interview by Lisa Gabbert, November 5, 2019. Salt Lake City, UT.

Gabbert, Lisa. 2011. *Winter Carnival in a Western Town; Identity, Change, and the Good of the Community.* Logan: Utah State University Press.

———. 2018. "Folk Drama." *Humanities* 7 (1). https://doi.org/10.3390/h7010002.

———. 2019. "American Festival and Folk Drama." In *The Oxford Handbook of American Folklore and Folklife Studies,* edited by Simon Bronner, 277–97. Oxford: Oxford University Press.

———. 2019–2020. Doctoring: The Occupational Folklore of Physicians: Archie Green Fellows Project. 2019–2020. AFC 2019/030: 05660. Archive of Folk Culture, American Folklife Center, Library of Congress, Washington, DC. https://www.loc.gov/collections/occupational-folklifeproject/?fa=partof:doctoring:+the+occupational+folklore+of+physicians:+archie+green+fellows+project,+2019-2020.

———. 2020. "Suffering in Medical Contexts: Laughter, Humor, and the Medical Carnivalesque." *Journal of American Folklore* 133 (527): 3–26. muse.jhu.edu/article/745701.

———. 2023. "Humor in the Time of Pandemic: Coronavirus and Expert Health Knowledge." Special issue, *Journal of Folklore Research* 60 (1): 43–58.

Gabbert, Lisa, and Anton Salud. 2009. "On Slanderous Words and Bodies Out-of-Control: Hospital Humor and the Medical Carnivalesque." In *The Body in Medical Culture*, edited by Elizabeth Klaver, 209–27. Albany: State University of New York Press.

Gambino, Matthew. 2013. "Erving Goffman's *Asylums* and Institutional Culture in the Mid-Twentieth-Century United States." *Harvard Review of Psychiatry* 21 (1): 52–57. https://doi.org/10.1097/HRP.0b013e31827d7df4.

George, Victoria, and Alan Dundes. 1978. "The Gomer: A Figure of American Hospital Folk Speech." *Journal of American Folklore* 91 (359): 568–81. https://doi.org/10.2307/539575.

Giddens, Anthony. 1990. *The Consequences of Modernity*. Stanford, CA: Stanford University Press.

Gibbs, Mary. 2019. Recorded interview by Lisa Gabbert, September 7, 2019. Salt Lake City, UT.

Glaser, Gabrielle. 2015. "Unfortunately, Doctors Are Pretty Good at Suicide." *Journal of Medicine*. August 15, 2015. ncnp.org/journal-of-medicine/1601-unfortunately-doctors-are-pretty-good-at-suicide.html.

Goffman, Erving. 1961. *Asylums: Essays on the Social Situation of Mental Patients and Other Inmates*. Garden City, NY: Anchor Books.

Gold, Jessica. 2011. "Cancer in the Gross Anatomy Lab." KevinMD.com. June 2, 2011. https://www.kevinmd.com/blog/2011/06/cancer-gross-anatomy-lab.html.

Gold, Katherine J., Ananda Sen, and Thomas L. Schwenk. 2013. "Details on Suicide among US Physicians: Data from the National Violent Death Reporting System." *General Hospital Psychiatry* 35 (1): 45–49. https://doi.org/10.1016/j.genhosppsych.2012.08.005.

Goldman, Dr. Brian. 2014. *The Secret Language of Doctors: Cracking the Code of Hospital Culture*. Chicago: Triumph Books.

Goldstein, Diane E. 2004. *Once Upon a Virus: AIDS Legends and Vernacular Risk Perception*. Logan: Utah State University Press.

GomerBlog (@GomerBlog). n.d. "Graduating Colorectal Fellow Realizes She Hates Poop." Pinterest pin. Accessed July 10, 2023. https://ar.pinterest.com/pin/483011128777153115/.

Gomerpedia. n.d. "American Academy of Orthopedic Surgeons." Accessed June 26, 2021. http://gomerpedia.org/wiki/American_Academy_of_Orthopaedic_Surgeons.

———. n.d. "Anesthesiology." Accessed June 26, 2021. http://gomerpedia.org/wiki/Category:Anesthesiology.

———. n.d. "Death." Accessed July 27, 2020. http://gomerpedia.org/wiki/Death.

———. n.d. "Psychiatry and Psychology." Accessed July 27, 2020. http://gomerpedia.org/wiki/Category:Psychiatry_%26_Psychology.

Gordon, David Paul. 1983. "Hospital Slang for Patients: Crocks, Gomers, Gorks, and Others." *Language in Society* 12 (2): 173–85. https://www.jstor.org/stable/4167396.

Graefer, Anne, Allaina Kilby, and Inger-Lise Kalviknes Bore. 2019. "Unruly Women and Carnivalesque Countercountrol: Offensive Humor in Mediated Social Protest." *Journal of Communication Inquiry* 43 (2): 171–93. https://doi.org/10.1177/0196859918800485.

Grayson, W. Paul. 1981. "The Folklore of a Medical Community." *Louisiana Folklore Miscellany* 5 (1): 48–52.

Green, Archie. 1987. "At the Hall, In the Stope: Who Treasures Tales of Work?" *Western Folklore* 46 (3): 153–70.

Groce, Nancy. 2010. *Lox, Stocks, and Backstage Broadway: Iconic Trades of New York City*. Washington, DC: Smithsonian Institution Scholarly Press.

———. 2019. "American Occupational Folklife: Work, Workers, and Workscapes." In *The Oxford Handbook of American Folklore and Folklife Studies*, edited by Simon J. Bronner, 825–44. Oxford: Oxford University Press.

Grow, Brian, and John Shiffman. 2017. "In the U.S. Market for Human Bodies, Almost Anyone Can Dissect and Sell the Dead." October 24, 2017. *Reuters Investigates*. Part of "The Body Trade" series. https://www.reuters.com/investigates/special-report/usa-bodies-brokers/.

Gupta, Rahul, Daniele R. Nolan, Donald A. Bux, and Andres R. Schneeberger. 2019. "Is It the Moon? Effects of the Lunar Cycle on Psychiatric Admissions, Discharges, and Length of Stay." *Swiss Medical Weekly*, April 23, 149 (1718):w20070. https://doi.org/10.4414/smw.2019.20070.

Hafferty, Frederic W. 1988. "Cadaver Stories and the Emotional Socialization of Medical Students." *Journal of Health and Social Behavior* 29 (4): 344–56. https://doi.org/10.2307/2136868.

———. 1991. *Into the Valley: Death and the Socialization of Medical Students*. New Haven, CT: Yale University Press.

Hancock, Dene, Maynard Williams, Antony Taylor, and Brenda Dawson. 2004. "Impact of Cadaver Dissection on Medical Students." *New Zealand Journal of Psychology* 33 (1): 17–25.

Hand, Wayland D. n.d. The Wayland D. Hand Collection of Superstition and Popular Belief. Folk Collection 36, Fife Folklore Archives, Special Collections and Archives, Utah State University.

———. 1980. *Magical Medicine: The Folkloric Component of Medicine in the Folk Belief, Custom, and Ritual of the Peoples of Europe and America*. Berkeley: University of California Press.

Harvard Medical School. 2021–2022. "Facts and Figures: HMS by the Numbers, FY2022." July 1, 2021–June 30, 2022. https://hms.harvard.edu/about-hms/facts-figures.

Hem, Erlend, Tor Haldorsen, Olaf Gjerløw Aasland, Reidar Tyssen, Per Vaglum, and Oivind Ekeberg. 2005. "Suicide Rates according to Education with a

Particular Focus on Physicians in Norway 1960–2000." *Psychological Medicine* 35 (6): 873–80. https://doi.org/10.1017/s0033291704003344.

Ho, Karen. 2009. *Liquidated: An Ethnography of Wall Street.* Durham, NC: Duke University Press Books.

Hochberg, Mark S. 2007. "The Doctor's White Coat: An Historical Perspective." *AMA Journal of Ethics* 9 (4): 310–14. https://doi.org/10.1001/virtualmentor.2007.9.4.mhst1-0704.

Hoffman, Matt, and Kevin Kunzmann. 2018. "Suffering in Silence: The Scourge of Physician Suicide." *HCPLive*, February 05, 2018. https://www.hcplive.com/view/suffering-in-silence-the-scourge-of-physician-suicide#.

Horlacher, Stefan. 2009. "A Short Introduction to Theories of Humour, the Comic, and Laughter." In *Gender and Laughter: Comic Affirmation and Subversion in Traditional and Modern Media,* edited by Gaby Pailer, Andreas Böhn, Stefan Horlacher, and Ulrich Scheck, 17–47. Albuquerque: University of New Mexico Press.

Houck, Anita. 2007. "The Ambiguous Laughter of Reconcilliation: Comic Theodicy in Modern Literature." *Religion and Literature* 39 (1) 47–78.

Howell, Joel D. 2016. "A History of Medical Residency." *Reviews in American History* 44 (1): 126–31.

Hufford, David. 1989. "Customary Observances in Modern Medicine." *Western Folklore* 48 (2): 129–43.

———. 1998. "Folklore Studies Applied to Health." *Journal of Folklore Research* 35 (3): 295–313.

Iacobucci, Gareth. 2019. "GP Suicides: LMCs Call for Action to Reduce 'Appalling' Numbers." *BMJ* 364:I1286. https://doi.org/10.1136/bmj.I1286.

Indiana University School of Medicine. 2022–2023. "Fact Sheet." Accessed May 16, 2023. https://mc-42b990dd-5dae-4647-b81e-424724-cdn-endpoint.azureedge.net/-/media/files/iusm-fact-sheet.pdf?rev=0a86ddfb2c3945daaab48259ed439c6d.

Ingram, Karen. 2020. Recorded interview by Lisa Gabbert, February 13, 2020. Salt Lake City, UT.

Jansen, William Hugh. 1959. "The Esoteric-Exoteric Factor in Folklore." *Fabula* 2 (2): 205–11. https://doi.org/10.1515/fabl.1959.2.2.205.

Joeckel, Samuel. 2008. "Funny as Hell: Christianity and Humor Reconsidered." *Humor: International Journal of Humor Research* 21 (4): 415–33.

Jones, Michael Owen 1994. "A Folklorist's Approach to Organizational Behavior (OB) and Organizational Development (OD)." In *Putting Folklore to Use,* edited by Michael Owen Jones, 162–86. Lexington: University Press of Kentucky.

Kahn, David L., and Richard H. Steeves. 1994. "Witnesses to Suffering: Nursing Knowledge, Voice, and Vision." *Nursing Outlook* 42 (6): 260–64.

Kane, Leslie. 2021. "'Death by 1000 Cuts': Medscape National Physician Burnout, Depression & Suicide Report 2021." *Medscape Internal Medicine*, January 22, 2021. https://www.medscape.com/slideshow/2021-lifestyle-burnout-6013456#2.

Katritzky, M. A. 2001. "Marketing Medicine: The Image of the Early Modern Mountebank." *Renaissance Studies* 15 (2): 121–53.

Kay, Adam. 2017. *This Is Going to Hurt: Secret Diaries of a Medical Resident*. New York: Little, Brown Spark.

Kazantzidis, George. 2018. "Doctors in a Comic Costume: Medical Language and Mass Audience in the Comedy of Menander." *Illinois Classical Studies* 43 (1): 25–57.

Kelly, Suzanne. 2012. "Dead Bodies That Matter: Toward a New Ecology of Human Death in American Culture." *Journal of American Culture* 35 (1): 37–50.

Kitta, Andrea. 2012. *Vaccinations and Public Concern in History: Legend, Rumor, and Risk Perception*. New York: Routledge.

Kleinman, A., and J. Kleinman. 1991. "Suffering and Its Professional Transformation: Toward an Ethnography of Interpersonal Experience." *Culture, Medicine and Psychiatry* 15 (3): 275–301.

Koch, Gertraud. 2012. "Work and Professions." In *A Companion to Folklore*, edited by Regina F. Bendix and Galit Hasan-Rokem, 154–68. Malden, MA: Wiley-Blackwell.

Korsmeyer, Carolyn. 2002. "Delightful, Delicious, Disgusting." *Journal of Aesthetics and Art Criticism* 60 (3): 217–25.

Kruesi, Margaret. 2004. "Herbs! Roots! Barks! Leaves!" *Folklife Center News* 26 (4): 5–7.

Kvideland, Reimund, and Hennig K. Sehmsdorf, eds. 1988. *Scandinavian Folk Belief and Legend*. Minneapolis: University of Minnesota Press.

Lachmann, Renate. 1988–89. "Bakhtin and Carnival: Culture as Counter-Culture." Translated by Raoul Eshelman and Marc Davis. *Cultural Critique* 11:115–52. https://doi.org/10.2307/1354246

Laudun, John. 2023. "Weathering the Storm: Folk Ideas about Character." In *Wait Five Minutes: Weatherlore in the Twenty-First Century*, edited by Shelley Ingram and Willow G. Mullins, 226–47. Jackson: University Press of Mississippi.

Lawton, Ashka. 2020. Recorded interview by Lisa Gabbert, July 21, 2020. Salt Lake City, UT.

Leary, James P. 2013. "Introduction: Class War and Laborlore." *Western Folklore* 72 (3–4): 316–20.

Lee, Jon D. 2014. *An Epidemic of Rumors: How Stories Shape Our Perceptions of Disease*. Logan: Utah State University Press.

Lintott, Sheila. 2016. "Superiority in Humor Theory." *Journal of Aesthetics and Art Criticism* 74 (4): 347–58.

Livingston, Paisley N. 1979. "Comic Treatment: Molière and the Farce of Medicine." *MLN* 94 (4): 676–87. https://doi.org/10.2307/2906292.

Lloyd-Jones, Hugh. 1971. "Menander's 'Aspis.'" *Greek, Roman, and Byzantine Studies* 12:175–95.

Longsworth, Robert. 1971. "The Doctor's Dilemma: A Comic View of the 'Physician's Tale.'" *Criticism* 13 (3): 223–33.

Low, Hana. 2010. "Letter to the other side." KevinMD.com (blog), May 7, 2010. http://www.kevinmd.com/blog/2010/05/medical-student-writes-gross-anatomy-cadaver.html.

Ludmerer, Kenneth M. 2014. *Let Me Heal: The Opportunity to Preserve Excellence in American Medicine.* Oxford: Oxford University Press.

Lupton, Deborah. 2003. *Medicine as Culture.* 2nd ed. London: Sage Publications.

Marsh, Moira. 2015. *Practically Joking.* Logan: Utah State University Press.

———. 2019. "American Jokes, Pranks, and Humor." In *The Oxford Handbook of American Folklore and Folklife Studies,* edited by Simon Bronner, 210–37. Oxford: Oxford University Press.

Maslach, Christina, and Michael P. Leiter. 2016. "Understanding the Burnout Experience: Recent Research and Its Implications for Psychiatry." *World Psychiatry* 15 (2): 103–11. https://doi.org/10.1002/wps.20311.

Massey, Susan. 2019. Recorded interview by Lisa Gabbert, November 5, 2019. Salt Lake City, UT.

McCarl, Robert. 1978. "Occupational Folklife: A Theoretical Hypothesis." In *Working Americans: Contemporary Approaches to Occupational Folklife,* edited by Robert H. Byington, 3–18. Los Angeles: California Folklore Society.

———. 2006. "Foreword: Lessons of Work and Workers." *Western Folklore* 65 (1–2): 13–29.

McClean, Sean. 2020. Recorded interview by Lisa Gabbert, February 24, 2020. Salt Lake City, UT.

McCrary, S., and R. C. Christensen. 1993. "Slang 'On Board': A Moral Analysis of Medical Jargon." *Archives of Family Medicine* 2 (1): 101–5. https://doi.org/10.1001/archfami.2.1.101.

McCreaddie, May, and Sally Wiggins. 2008. "The Purpose and Function of Humour in Health, Health Care and Nursing: A Narrative Review." *Journal of Advanced Nursing* 61 (6): 584–95. doi: 10.1111/j.1365-2648.2007.04548.x

McDonald, Steven. 2020. "No One Is Supporting the Doctors." *The Atlantic,* April 18, 2020. https://www.theatlantic.com/ideas/archive/2020/04/doctors-already-manage-alone/610249/.

McHoul, Alec, and Wendy Grace. 1997. *A Foucault Primer: Discourse, Power and the Subject.* New York: New York University Press.

McLay, Robert N., Amado A. Daylo, and Paul S. Hammer. 2006. "No Effect of Lunar Cycle on Psychiatric Admissions or Emergency Evaluations." *Military Medicine* 171 (12): 1239–42.

McNamara, Brooks. 1984. "The Medicine Show Log: Reconstructing a Traditional American Entertainment." *Drama Review: TDR* 28 (3): 74–97.

Mechling, Jay. 2019. "Total Institutions: Camps, Boarding Schools, Military Bases, Hospitals, and Prisons in American Folklore and Folklife." In *Oxford Handbook of American Folklore and Folklife*, edited by Simon Bronner, 669–87. Oxford: Oxford University Press.

Messybeast.com. n.d. "Doctors' Slang, Medical Slang and Medical Acronyms and Veterinary Acronyms & Vet Slang." Accessed July 6, 2023. http://messybeast .com/dragonqueen/medical-acronyms.htm.

Miller, Montana. 2012. *Playing Dead: Mock Trauma and Folk Drama in Staged High School Drunk Driving Tragedies*. Logan: Utah State University Press.

Mirhosseini, Seyyed-Abdolhamid, and Hossein Fattahi. 2010. "The Language of 'Circule': Discursive Construction of False Referral in Iranian Teaching Hospitals." *Medical Anthropology Quarterly* 24 (3): 304–25. https://doi.org/10.1111 /j.1548-1387.2010.01106.x.

Mitford, Jessica. 1963. *The American Way of Death*. New York: Simon and Schuster.

Mizrahi, Terry. 1986. *Getting Rid of Patients: Contradictions in the Socialization of Physicians*. New Brunswick, NJ: Rutgers University Press.

Montell, William Lynwood. 2008. *Tales from Kentucky Doctors*. Lexington: University Press of Kentucky.

Moore, Jamie. 1991. "Poetry, Puns, and Pediatrics: The Verbal Artistry of Dr. James L. Hughes." *North Carolina Folklore Journal* 38 (1): 45–71.

Morris, Pam, ed. 1994. *The Bakhtin Reader: Selected Writings of Bakhtin, Medvedev, and Voloshinov*. London: Arnold.

Morse, Gardiner. 2010. "Health Care Needs a New Kind of Hero." Edited interview with Atul Gawande. *Harvard Business Review*, April 2010. https://hbr.org /2010/04/health-care-needs-a-new-kind-of-hero.

Moxham, Bernard J., and Odile Plaisant. 2014. "The History of the Teaching of Gross Anatomy—How We Got to Where We Are!" *European Journal of Anatomy* 18 (3): 219–44.

Mullen, Patrick. 2000. "Belief and the American Folk." *Journal of American Folklore* 113 (448): 119–43. http://www.jstor.org/stable/541285.

Narváez, Peter, ed. 2003. *Of Corpse: Death and Humor in Folklore and Popular Culture*. Logan: Utah State University Press.

911doc. 2008. "The 'O,' 'Q ,' and 'Dotted Q' Signs." *M.D.O.D.*, June 6, 2008. http:// docsontheweb.blogspot.com/2008/06/o-q-and-dotted-q-signs.html.

Noseworthy, John, James Madara, Delos Cosgrove, Mitchell Edgeworth, Ed Ellison, Sarah Krevans, Paul Rothman, et al. 2017. "Physician Burnout Is a Public Health Crisis: A Message to Our Fellow Health Care CEOs." *Health Affairs*, March 28, 2017 . https://www.healthaffairs.org/content/forefront

/physician-burnout-public-health-crisis-message-our-fellow-health
-care-ceos.

Nutton, Vivian. 2001. "God, Galen, and the Depaganization of Ancient Medicine." In *Religion and Medicine in the Middle Ages*, edited by Peter Biller and
Joseph Ziegler, 15–32. Suffolk, UK: York Medieval Press.

NYU Langone Health. 2019. "The Making of the House of God." July 10, 2019.
JAMA Network. 26 min 53 sec. https://edhub.ama-assn.org/jn-learning/video
-player/17710195.

Obrdlik, Antonin J. 1942. "'Gallows Humor'—A Sociological Phenomenon."
American Journal of Sociology 47 (5): 709–16.

O'Connor, Bonnie Blair. 1995. *Healing Traditions: Alternative Medicine and the
Health Professions*. Philadelphia: University of Pennsylvania Press.

Odean, Kathleen. 1995. "Anal Folklore in the Medical World." In *Folklore Interpreted: Essays in Honor of Alan Dundes*, edited by Regina Bendix and Rosemary
Lévy Zumwalt, 137–52. New York: Garland Publishing.

Oreskovich, Michael R., Krista L. Kaups, Charles M. Balch, John B. Hanks, Daniel
Satele, Jeff Sloan, Charles Meredith, Amanda Buhl, Lotte N. Dyrbye, and Tait D.
Shanafelt. 2012. "Prevalence of Alcohol Use Disorders among American Surgeons."
Archives of Surgery 147 (2): 168–74. https://doi.org/10.1001/archsurg.2011.1481.

Oring, Elliott. 2008. *Engaging Humor*. Urbana: University of Illinois Press.

———. 2008. "Legendry and the Rhetoric of Truth." *Journal of American Folklore*
121 (480): 127–66.

———. 2011. "Parsing the Joke: The General Theory of Verbal Humor and Appropriate Incongruity." *Humor: International Journal of Humor Research* 24 (2):
203–22.

Osborne, Thomas. 1994. "On Anti-Medicine and Clinical Reason." In *Reassessing
Foucault: Power, Medicine and the Body*, edited by Colin Jones and Roy Porter,
28–47. London: Routledge.

Outram, Sue, and Brian Kelly. 2014. "'You Teach Us to Listen, . . . But You Don't
Teach Us about Suffering': Self-Care and Resilience Strategies in Medical
School Curricula." *Perspectives on Medical Education* 3:371–78.

Pai, Anushka, Alina M. Suris, and Carol S. North. 2017. "Posttraumatic Stress
Disorder in the DSM-5: Controversy, Change, and Conceptual Considerations." *Behavioral Sciences* 7 (1): 7. https://doi.org/10.3390/bs7010007.

Parsons, G. N., S. B. Kinsman, C. L. Bosk, P. Sankar, and P. A. Ubel. 2001. "Between Two Worlds: Medical Student Perceptions of Humor and Slang in the
Hospital Setting." *Journal of General Internal Medicine* 16 (8): 544–49. https://
doi.org/10.1046/j.1525-1497.2001.016008544.x.

Parsons, Talcott. 1951. "Illness and the Role of the Physician: A Sociological Perspective."
American Journal of Orthopsychiatry 21 (3): 452–60. https://onlinelibrary.wiley
.com/doi/10.1111/j.1939-0025.1951.tb00003.x.

Paz, Octavio. 1961. *The Labyrinth of Solitude: Life and Thought in Mexico*. Translated by Lysander Kemp. New York: Grove Press.

Penn Medicine News. 2019. "Minority Students Still Underrepresented in Medical School." News release, September 4, 2019. https://www.pennmedicine.org /news/news-releases/2019/september/minority-students-still-underrepresented -in-medical-schools.

Penson, Richard T., Rosamund A. Partridge, Pandora Rudd, Michael V. Seiden, Jill E. Nelson, Bruce A. Chabner, and Thomas J. Lynch. 2005. "Update: Laughter: The Best Medicine?" *The Oncologist* 10 (8): 651–60. https://doi.org/10.1634 /theoncologist.10-8-651.

Peterson, C. 1998. "Medical Slang in Rio de Janeiro, Basil." *Cadernos de Saúde Pública* 14 (4): 671–82.

Pound, Louise. 1936. "American Euphemisms for Dying, Death, and Burial: An Anthology." *American Speech* 11 (3): 195–202.

Prahlad, Anand. 2021. "Tearing Down Monuments: Missed Opportunities, Silences, and Absences—A Radical Look at Race in American Folklore Studies." *Journal of American Folklore* 134 (533): 258–64.

Price, Brian. 2019. Recorded interview by Lisa Gabbert, November 8, 2019. Salt Lake City, UT.

Radetsky, Michael. 2015. "The Hero in Medicine." *JAMA* 313 (17): 1715. https:// doi.org/10.1001/jama.2015.3390.

Ravenscroft, Neil, and Paul Gilchrist. 2009. "Spaces of Transgression: Governance, Discipline, and the Reworking of the Carnivalesque." *Leisure Studies* 28 (1): 35–49. https://doi.org/10.1080/02614360802127243.

Robbins, Roni. 2022. "Medscape Residents Salary & Debt Report 2022." Medscape, July 29, 2002. https://www.medscape.com/slideshow/2022-residents -salary-debt-report-6015490.

Reifler, Douglas R. 1996. "'I Don't Actually Mind the Bone Saw': Narratives of Gross Anatomy." *Literature and Medicine* 15 (2): 183–99. https://doi.org/10.1353 /lm.1996.0024.

Robertson, D. W. 1988. "The Physician's Comic Tale." *Chaucer Review* 23 (2): 129–39.

Rosenzweig, Steven. 1996. "The Physician as Hero." *Academic Emergency Medicine* 3 (6): 650. PMID: 8727639.

Roth, LuAnne. 2017. "'You Are What Others Think You Eat': Food, Identity, and Subjectivity in Zombie Protagonist Narratives." In *What's Eating You?: Food and Horror on Screen*, edited by Cynthia J. Miller and A. Bowdoin van Riper, 271–92. New York: Bloomsbury Academic.

Rudlin, John. 1994. *Commedia dell'Arte: An Actor's Handbook*. New York: Routledge.

Rundblad, Georganne. 1995. "Exhuming Women's Premarket Duties in the Care of the Dead." *Gender and Society* 9 (2): 173–92.

Russo, Mary. 1986. "Female Grotesques: Carnival and Theory." In *Feminist Studies/ Critical Studies*, edited by Teresa de Lauretis, 213–29. Bloomington: Indiana University Press.

Samuel, Lawrence R. 2013. *Death, American Style: A Cultural History of Dying in America*. Lanham: Rowman and Littlefield.

Santino, Jack, ed. 2017. *Public Performances: Studies in the Carnivalesque and Ritualesque*. Logan: Utah State University Press.

Schmidt, Claire. 2017. *If You Don't Laugh, You'll Cry: The Occupational Humor of White Wisconsin Prison Workers*. Madison: University of Wisconsin Press.

Schrager, Samuel. 1999. *The Trial Lawyer's Art*. Philadelphia: Temple University Press.

Schuld, J., J. E. Slotta, S. Schuld, O. Kollmar, M. K. Schilling, and S. Richter. 2011. "Popular Belief Meets Surgical Reality: Impact of Lunar Phases, Friday the 13th and Zodiac Signs on Emergency Operations and Intraoperative Blood Loss." *World J Surgery* 35 (9): 1945–49. https://doi.org/10.1007/s00268 -011-1166-8.

Schulz, Max. 1973. "Toward a Definition of Black Humor." *The Southern Review* 1 (9): 117–34.

Schweikart, Scott J. 2020. "Could Humor in Health Care Become Malpractice?" *AMA Journal of Ethics* 22 (7): 596–601.

Scott, James C. 1998. *Seeing Like a State: How Certain Schemes to Improve the Human Condition Have Failed*. New Haven, CT: Yale University Press.

Segal, Daniel A. 1988. "A Patient So Dead: American Medical Students and Their Cadavers." *Anthropological Quarterly* 61 (1): 17–25. https://doi.org/10.2307 /3317868.

Selzer, Richard. 1975. "The Corpse." *Esquire*, May 1, 1975, 74–76.

Shanafelt, Tait D., Charles M. Balch, Lotte Dyrbye, Gerald Bechamps, Tom Russell, Daniel Satele, Teresa Rummans, et al. 2011. "Special Report: Suicidal Ideation among American Surgeons." *Archives of Surgery (Chicago, Ill.: 1960)* 146 (1): 54–62. https://doi.org/10.1001/archsurg.2010.292.

Shanafelt, Tait D., Sonja Boone, Litjen Tan, Lotte N. Dyrbye, Wayne Sotile, Daniel Satele, Colin P. West, Jeff Sloan, and Michael R. Oreskovich. 2012. "Burnout and Satisfaction with Work-Life Balance among US Physicians Relative to the General US Population." *Archives of Internal Medicine* 172 (18): 1377–85. https:// doi.org/10.1001/archinternmed.2012.3199.

Shanafelt, Tait D., Omar Hasan, Lotte N. Dyrbye, Christine Sinsky, Daniel Satele, Jeff Sloan, and Colin P. West. 2015. "Changes in Burnout and Satisfaction with Work-Life Balance in Physicians and the General US Working Population between 2011 and 2014." *Mayo Clinic Proceedings* 90 (12): 1600–1613. https://doi.org/10.1016/j.mayocp.2015.08.023.

Shem, Samuel. (1978) 2003. *The House of God*. New York: Delta Trade Paperbacks.

Sheppard, Will. 2019. Recorded interview by Lisa Gabbert, September 20, 2019. Salt Lake City, UT.

Singh, Dubb, S., A. Ferro, and C. Fowell. 2021. "'Shh—Don't Say the Q-Word' or Do You?" *British Journal of Oral and Maxillofacial Surgery* 59 (1): e13–e16. https://doi.org/10.1016/j.bjoms.2020.08.044.

Siporin, Steve. 2022. *The Befana Is Returning: The Story of a Tuscan Festival*. Madison: University of Wisconsin Press.

Skomorowsky, Anne. 2014. "Big Boobs Matter Most." *Pacific Standard*, October 20, 2014. Updated June 14, 2017. https://psmag.com/social-justice/medical-mnemonics-sexist-medicine-health-care-big-boobs-matter-most-92773.

Smedley, B. D., A. Stith Butler, and L. R. Bristow, eds. 2004. *In the Nation's Compelling Interest: Ensuring Diversity in the Health-Care Workforce*. Washington, DC: National Academies Press.

Smith, Moira. 2009. "Humor, Unlaughter, and Boundary Maintenance." *Journal of American Folklore* 122 (484): 148–71.

Sobel, Rachel K. 2006. "Does Laughter Make Good Medicine?" *New England Journal of Medicine* 354 (11): 1114–15.

Sotile, Wayne M. 2019. "RESPONSE: Time to End the Conspiracy of Silence about Physician Suffering." *Journal of the American College of Cardiology* 73 (4): 523–24. https://doi.org/10.1016/j.jacc.2018.12.021.

Spectator. 2017. "The Cult of the Prima Doctor." No. 6 (May). https://www.spectator.co.uk/article/the-cult-of-the-prima-doctor.

Sprunger, David A. 1996. "Parodic Animal Physicians from the Margins of Medieval Manuscripts." In *Animals in the Middle Ages*, edited by Nona C. Flores, 67–83. New York: Routledge.

Strauman, Elena C., and Bethany C. Goodier. 2011. "The Doctor(s) in House: An Analysis of the Evolution of the Television Doctor-Hero." *Journal of Medical Humanities* 32 (1): 31–46. https://doi.org/10.1007/s10912-010-9124-2.

Stukator, Angela. 2001. "'It's Not Over until the Fat Lady Sings': Comedy, the Carnivalesque, and Body Politics." In *Bodies Out of Bounds: Fatness and Transgression*, edited by Jana Evans Braziel and Kathleen LeBesco, 197–213. Berkeley: University of California Press.

Subramanian, P., S. Kantharuban, V. Subramanian, S. A. G. Willis-Owen, and C.A. Willis-Owen. 2011. "Orthopaedic Surgeons: As Strong as an Ox and Almost Twice as Clever? Multicentre Prospective Comparative Study." *BMJ* 343:d7506. https://doi.org/10.1136/bmj.d7506.

Symon, Robyn, director. 2018. *Do No Harm*. DCP. 85 min.

Take Aurally (@takeaurally5245). 2017. "Suman Biswas Performs 'Drugs Song' at Das SMACC." July 15, 2017. YouTube video, 2:24. https://www.youtube.com/watch?v=vkKZLODDOVs.

Talbot, Simon G., and Wendy Dean. 2018. "Physicians Aren't 'Burning Out': They're Suffering from Moral Injury." *Statnews*, July 26, 2018. https://www .statnews.com/2018/07/26/physicians-not-burning-out-they-are-suffering -moral-injury/.

Tangherlini, Timothy R. 1996. s.v., "Legend." In *American Folklore: An Encyclopedia*, edited by Jan Harold Brunvand, 915–19. New York: Garland Publishing.

———. 1998. *Talking Trauma: A Candid Look at Paramedics through Their Tradition of Tale-Telling*. Jackson: University Press of Mississippi.

Taviani, Ferdinando. 2018. "Knots and Doubleness: The Engine of the Commedia dell'Arte." In *Commedia dell'Arte in Context*, edited by Christopher B. Balme, Piermario Vescovo, and Daniele Vianello, 17–33. Cambridge: Cambridge University Press. https://doi.org/10.1017/9781139236331

Tazobactar (@tazobactar). 2010. "Orthopedia vs Anesthesia (Orthopaedics, Anaesthetics, Conversation)." July 23, 2010. YouTube video, 3:21. https://www .youtube.com/watch?v=3rTsvb2ef5k.

Thomas, Jeannie B. 1997. *Featherless Chickens, Laughing Women, and Serious Stories*. Charlottesville: University of Virginia Press.

Thorson, James A. 1993. "Did You Ever See a Hearse Go By? Some Thoughts on Gallows Humor." *Journal of American Culture* 16 (2): 17–24. https://doi.org /10.1111/j.1542-734X.1993.00017.x.

Thursby, Jacqueline S. 2006. *Funeral Festivals in America: Rituals for the Living*. Lexington: University Press of Kentucky.

Tilley, Carol. 2018. "Of Cornopleezeepi and Party Poopers: A Brief History of Physicians in Comics." *AMA Journal of Ethics* 20 (2): 188–94. https://doi.org /10.1001/journalofethics.2018.20.2.mhst1-1802.

Tolpin, Jeremy. 2018. "On the Other Side of Physician Burnout." *STAT* (blog), May 17, 2018. https://www.statnews.com/2018/05/17/physician-burnout -working-part-time/.

Toynbee, Arnold. 1968. "Changing Attitudes towards Death in the Modern Western World." In *Man's Concern with Death*, edited by Arnold Toynbee, A. Keith Mant, Ninian Smart, John Hinton, Simon Yudkin, Eric Rhode, Rosalind Heywood, and H. H. Price, 122–32. London: Hodder and Stoughton.

Trahant, Yvette L. 1981. "The Oral Tradition of the Physician." *Louisiana Folklore Miscellany* 5 (1): 38–47.

Tseng, Wei-Ting, and Ya-Ping Lin. 2016. "'Detached Concern' of Medical Students in a Cadaver Dissection Course: A Phenomenological Study." *Anatomical Sciences Education* 9 (3): 265–71. https://doi.org/10.1002/ase.1579.

Verghese, Abraham. 1998. *The Tennis Partner*. New York: Harper Perennial.

Voltaire. 1901. *The Works of Voltaire. A Contemporary Version*. Edited by John Morley. Translated by William F. Fleming. Vol. 8. New York: E. R. DuMont. http://www.gutenberg.org/files/35628/35628-h/35628-h.htm.

Wagner, Paul, and Steve Zeitlin. 1983. *Free Show Tonite*. Original format: 16mm. Film. 58 minutes. https://www.folkstreams.net/films/free-show-tonite.

Wallis, Faith, ed. 2010. *Medieval Medicine: A Reader*. Toronto: University of Toronto Press.

Walsh, William. 2012. Recorded interview by Lisa Gabbert, December 2, 2012. Salt Lake City, UT.

———. 2015. Recorded interview by Lisa Gabbert, February 15, 2015. Salt Lake City, UT.

Ware, Carolyn E. 2007. *Cajun Women and Mardi Gras: Reading the Rules Backward*. Urbana: University of Illinois Press.

Warner, Ian. 2020. Recorded interview by Lisa Gabbert, January 13, 2020. Salt Lake City, UT.

Watson, Katie. 2011. "Gallows Humor in Medicine." *Hastings Center Report* 41 (5): 37–45.

Wear, Delese, Julie M. Aultman, Joseph Zarconi, and Joseph D. Varley. 2009. "Derogatory and Cynical Humour Directed towards Patients: Views of Residents and Attending Doctors." *Medical Education* 43 (1): 34–41. doi:10.1111/j.1365-2923.2008.03171.x

Westwood, Robert I., and Allanah Johnston. 2013. "Humor in Organization: From Function to Resistance." *Humor* 26 (2): 219–47.

Wickberg, Daniel. 1998. *The Senses of Humor: Self and Laughter in Modern America*. Ithaca, NY: Cornell University Press.

Williams, Anna. 2018. "Addressing the Lack of Women in Orthopaedic Surgery." Northwestern Medicine Feinberg School of Medicine News Center. October 15, 2018. https://news.feinberg.northwestern.edu/2018/10/15/addressing-the -lack-of-women-in-orthopaedic-surgery/.

Williams, Austin D., Emily E. Greenwald, Rhonda L. Soricelli, and Dennis M. DePace. 2014. "Medical Students' Reactions to Anatomic Dissection and the Phenomenon of Cadaver Naming." *Anatomical Sciences Education* 7 (3): 169–80. https://doi.org/10.1002/ase.1391.

Williamson, A. M., and A. M. Feyer. 2000. "Moderate Sleep Deprivation Produces Impairments in Cognitive and Motor Performance Equivalent to Legally Prescribed Levels of Alcohol Intoxication." *Occupational and Environmental Medicine* 57 (10): 649–55. https://doi.org/10.1136/oem.57.10.649.

Winick, Stephen D. 2004. "'You Can't Kill Shit': Occupational Proverb and Metaphorical System among Young Medical Professionals." In *What Goes around Comes Around: The Circulation of Proverbs in Contemporary Life*, edited by Kimberly J. Lau, Peter Tokofsky, and Stephen D. Winick, 86–106. Logan: Utah State University Press.

Wright, Joe. 2005. "Medical School, in and out of Anatomy Lab." NPR's *All Things Considered*, November 15, 2005. https://www.npr.org/2005 /11/15/5014042/medical-school-in-and-out-of-anatomy-lab.

Yasin, Meira Mahmoud. 2018. "From Syrian Refugee to Dishwasher to Heart Doctor: The Inspirational Story of Hero and Humanitarian Dr. Heval Kelli." *Journal of Health Care for the Poor and Underserved* 29 (1): 1–4. https://doi.org /10.1353/hpu.2018.0000.

Yoder, Don. 1972. "Folk Medicine." In *Folklore and Folklife: An Introduction*, edited by Richard Dorson, 191–215. Chicago: University of Chicago Press.

York, Mark. 2018. Recorded interview by Lisa Gabbert, September 6, 2018. Salt Lake City, UT.

Young, Katharine. 1997. *Presence in the Flesh: The Body in Medicine.* Cambridge, MA: Harvard University Press.

Zatta, Claudia. 2001. "Democritus and Folly: The Two Wise Fools." *Bibliothèque d'Humanisme et Renaissance* 63 (3): 533–49.

Zimdars, Melissa. 2015. "Fat Acceptance TV?: Rethinking Reality Television with TLC's *Big Sexy* and the Carnivalesque." *Popular Communication* 13 (3): 232–46. https://doi.org/10.1080/15405702.2015.1048344.

INDEX

Lisa Gabbert is Professor of English at Utah State University. She is author of *Winter Carnival in a Western Town: Identity, Change, and the Good of the Community* and (with Keiko Wells) of *An Introduction to Vernacular Culture in America: Society, Region, and Tradition.*

Antonio Salud II, MD, MA, is Pulmonary and Critical Care Medicine Physician at Ascension of Wisconsin and Assistant Clinical Professor at the Medical College of Wisconsin. He is coauthor with Lisa Gabbert of the article "On Slanderous Words and Bodies Out-of-Control: Hospital Humor and the Medical Carnivalesque."

For Indiana University Press

Lesley Bolton, Project Manager/Editor
Allison Chaplin, Acquisitions Editor
Anna Garnai, Editorial Assistant
Sophia Hebert, Assistant Acquisitions Editor
Samantha Heffner, Marketing and Publicity Manager
Brenna Hosman, Production Coordinator
Katie Huggins, Production Manager
Dan Pyle, Online Publishing Manager
Pamela Rude, Senior Artist and Book Designer